Symmetry:
The Physics of Pain

An introduction to Postural Alignment Technology™

Marlene! You are awesome for going through this program. Be proud of yourself + stay motivated!!

Written by Patrick R. Mummy

©Symmetry for Health - Patrick R. Mummy. All rights reserved. No part of this book may be used or reproduced in any manner whatsoever without written permission, except in case of brief quotations embodied in critical articles and reviews.

For more information e-mail all inquiries to: info@symmetryforhealth.com

ISBN# 978-0-692-08490-8

Printed in the USA

Dedication

I debated heavily whether to write a dedication in this book or not. In the end, I choose this simple gesture in order to publicly acknowledge those who have co-piloted my journey. It means a lot to me to recognize the people who have stayed the course, believing in me and in what I have created. Without them, the journey would have been very different, to say the least.

My late wife Lauren was inspiration personified. Her pedigree as a writer, story-teller, motivator, mother, friend, business partner and wife, was as good as it gets. I remember her waking up next to me one morning in 2002; she looked at me and said, "You can create something huge with this business, darling. All you have to do is write it down, and you will succeed." I did, and I have. Even during that fateful trip she took to South Africa, she was creating bigger plans for us upon her return. She will always be remembered.

My current wife Tricia carried me on her shoulders for longer than most would dare. Perhaps the strongest woman I know, she dealt with fall-out of war like proportions. She has always been my biggest champion, through thick and thin, and through it all, she enabled me to find my legs again, cheering me every step of the way. It will be a pleasure sharing this success with her for the rest of our lives.

To my children Ryenne, Jaide, Eric and Rachael. Two by gift, and two by choice. Life is defined by the family you have, and the family you choose. We were lucky enough to blend a beautiful mixture of crazy with talent, which has equaled love from the get-go. If your children aren't motivation enough to reach your level of desired inspiration, then I don't know what is.

To my business partners and best friends, both former and present. I met Michael, who was my first investor, as a client. When he was 19, he broke his neck cliff-diving off Sunset Cliffs in San Diego. He proved the doctors wrong 4 months later by walking again. I met him 26 years later when his injury had started to take its toll. He made such great progress with Symmetry that he invested in my first software program and we became fast friends. He was a true beacon of light. Andrew Duenas, a retired Air Force Chief Master Sergeant, who had everything in life to pursue after he retired, but chose to join Symmetry and share his vast expertise and knowledge with us. His unwavering support to our cause has been nothing short of sanctimony. Andy Rocklin: I fixed his knee; he fixed my life. I have never in my short time on this planet met someone as humble as he is, as willing to jump in at a moment's notice, give advice if asked, and never complain about his return on investment, or lack thereof! The man is patient.

What I love about what I do, and what I have created, is that over the 22 years I have been knee-deep into this field, I have met people that I can honestly call great friends and mentors. I was thinking about how many people I have evaluated and met over these years, and came up with nearly 7000. People like Az, who I watched play at San Diego State and for my Rams, winning a Super Bowl. Tony Gwynn, who flew me out to Peoria during Spring Training when he was a Padre, Steve

Emtman who forced me to train him in Symmetry when I still didn't have a clue. There are so many other athletes and celebrities I have been able to straighten out. Nonetheless, those I am the most honored to know and work with are all the clients that come in to Symmetry, willing to change their lives and take control of their future. People like the Sainz, who I love and adore. The Felds who I have maintained a friendship with for nearly 22 years, and who keep coming back for check-ups. Bill Randoll who has never stopped believing in me. These and all my clients are the people I dedicate this book to, because changing a paradigm doesn't come from a method. It comes from the countless number of supporters who believe that the system can change one person at a time.

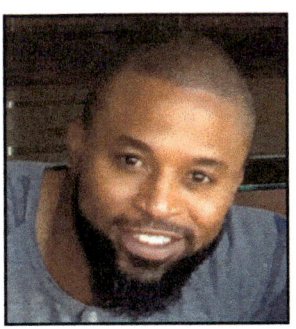

Forward written by Az Hakim

I want to let as many people know about Symmetry as possible, although many people are slow to warm up to new ideas when they don't know enough about something to truly value it. I know Symmetry changes lives, because it changed mine, and I know, once people witness with their own bodies how incredibly effective this technology is, they will value it indefinitely.

Patrick Mummy and I met back in 2005 when I was working with a trainer named Harland Svare. During the off-season, Harland worked to prepare me for the rigorous battles of the NFL. One day while training with several partners who were already battling injuries, a friend of mine began experiencing back issues that prevented him from working out. Harland, seeing my partner injured and in pain, decided to schedule an appointment to take us to Patrick's office in La Jolla. We didn't even practice that morning, we just went straight to his office.

I remember shaking his hand. When I introduced myself, Patrick's eyes lit up. As it turned out, he had been a fan of mine for quite some time: he followed my career from the time I played at his Alma Mater as well, San Diego State University, until I played for the St. Louis Ram's and won a Super Bowl championship in 2000. We had very parallel lives but never connected until this day.

From the very beginning, Patrick and I hit it off. He told me about his company and what he does and assured me that if I ever needed him he would be there for me. I knew immediately that he was a man of his word and I could rely on him. Looking back now, I should've taken the initiative right there on the spot to go through a routine, but, since I wasn't necessarily hurting at the time—and didn't understand that this technology would help me regardless—I wasn't able to fully reap the benefits of our first introduction.

In 2005 I went to a training camp with the New Orleans Saints. It was the year of Hurricane Katrina so our training took place in San Antonio, Texas. At practice one day I broke a tackle and immediately tried to accelerate after spinning off one of my teammates. Being that my body wasn't in alignment, and because of my attempt to accelerate from the position I was in, I pulled my hamstring. I was out for six weeks before I was even able to participate and practice fully with my teammates.

I knew I had to do something. Even more, I knew that the traditional methods of help were not doing enough to get me back up to speed and back in the game. I would get a treatment and be asked how I was feeling each time, then be sent out prematurely only to reinjure my hamstring. This happened to me three times before I realized what I was missing.

I called Patrick and flew him out to San Antonio. Once we were together, Patrick immediately took my measurements. He told me one hip was elevated six degrees higher than the other and rotated forward, and then explained this was the main reason I was experiencing problems. I was astounded. I laughed at him, "Yeah, go figure!" However, after taking my measurements, Patrick then created and took me through my first sequence of corrective exercises.

After leading me through my routine he asked me to walk and then jog. I didn't feel any hamstring tightness or tension in my long-gate. I was amazed at the benefits I *immediately* received from his technology. And I was impressed. I was on the field the next day practicing with my teammates, and I never struggled with my hamstring again. Experiencing the restoration of my abilities after not being able to train a single day for the previous six weeks made me realize his technology was a game-changer. In that moment, I became an official believer in Patrick and in Symmetry.

Integrating Symmetry's Postural Alignment Technology™ into my daily routine did tremendous wonders for my being—both my body and my soul—because I was able to think more clearly. Through the process of realigning my body something amazing happened. It seemed the technology not only aligned my body, but prepared me mentally for each day. For the first time, I felt aligned physically *and* spiritually. I noticed I was able to focus longer, think more clearly, push myself physically without fear of injury, and I no longer experienced kinks in my neck that I periodically had after a night of sleeping crookedly. Most days, after completing my routine, I discovered the remainder of my day flowed in such a way that I was able to achieve whatever I had set out for the day. I was determined to continue my routine throughout (and beyond) the rest of my NFL career. It has helped me tremendously both professionally and personally. This program, in many ways, changed my life.

I wasn't the only one to experience these incredible results. My family went through Symmetry as well. My father, who struggled with back issues and lethargy was able to alleviate his back pain altogether while simultaneously increasing his energy levels. All while the doctors continued to recommend surgery.

My teammates noticed a shift, too. While I was going through Symmetry, Patrick was also working with a few teammates of mine, Ernie Conwell and Steve Gleason to name a couple, and these guys were very invested in taking care of their bodies. They knew Patrick was on to something when he worked with them and their alignment. It takes extreme skill to know what is wrong with your body, how to identify the problem, and then to take an isometric exercise and use it to rebuild your body. This knowledge was key to us.

One day while Patrick and I were meeting he mentioned one of my teammates—Deuce McAllister—to me. Patrick told me, quite vehemently, that he wanted me to speak to Deuce on his behalf, and asked me to bring him in. Patrick believed he was favoring his right leg. I found this assessment odd because I knew Deuce didn't have any knee or leg problems at the time. Regardless, Patrick believed Deuce was on the precipice of a serious injury due to how severely he was favoring his right leg, and he believed his technology could help if he was given the chance to meet with him.

Two weeks later Patrick came to visit me to see how my body was responding to the corrective routine. When I saw him, I immediately asked him how he could have possibly predicted Deuce's knee injury. Patrick hadn't even known, but in between trips, Deuce had suffered a severe right-knee injury, an injury that he incurred without ever coming into contact with another player. And Patrick said it was going to happen! It was an unfortunate accident that Patrick had been trying to get Deuce to avoid, though he never got the opportunity.

An incredible toll is placed on your body when you play a high-performance sport competitively, and athletes need to understand there is life after sports. Symmetry is designed to help at any stage of a competitive athletic career: before, during, and after. The reality, however, is that *so many people wait until they are in pain to do something about it*. What most people don't realize is the empowerment in and importance of taking preventative measures to ensure your body stays healthy in all circumstances.

An even bigger reality, which is the reason Postural Alignment Technology™ is having such a difficult time breaking into the professional and sports arena, is that people are scared of the new and of what they don't know. Quite frankly, implementing Symmetry's Postural Alignment Technology™ into the sports medicine arena would leave a lot of people without jobs. The trainers who assess sports injury rely heavily on players to continue getting injured in order to maintain job security. It's an ugly truth that needs to be said: if injuries were being addressed at the cause (rather than the effect) a large number of sports medicine trainers would be out of a job. Instead, these trainers and people in high-powered positions continue handing athlete's old remedies such as "ice and stim," and "rest is best." However, if your body isn't in proper alignment then the therapy you receive never has the chance to address the root of the problem, and therefore your body is never able to fully recover. This explains why so many athletes become injured, go through typical therapy protocols, recuperate, are injured shortly after recuperating, and the cycle continues. The effect, rather than the cause of pain, is being treated. Symmetry is the first method I know of that doesn't treat symptoms: it addresses the cause of pain, removing the symptoms altogether.

It's extremely important for high performance businesses, with athletes playing at the highest levels, and where competitive sports place a great demand on an athlete's body, to find a form of therapy that works—particularly where professional athletes are concerned. Instead, injury is the new lifestyle. People would rather wake up and ice an ankle than wake up with a routine, simply because it is what they are used to. Nevertheless, if you're not waking up with a routine—and actively seeking to get your body in proper alignment—your body's compensation patterns will eventually wear you down, and injury will arise again and again- regardless of whether you are a professional athlete, or not.

My hope is to communicate to all higher-ups, both in the professional sports arena and the healthcare arena, that Symmetry defines the new format of training and performance. Bringing your body into proper and maximized alignment is the most efficient and effective way for one to take their performance to the next level. When a person aligns their body, they are better equipped and able to focus on a rigorous workout. It is because of this that Symmetry belongs in every sport, in every college program, in every gym, sports medicine and physical therapy book, and certainly in every home: if you're playing a sport, Symmetry needs to be implemented into your daily routine; if you are a coach, your players need to have these routines; if you maintain a sports medicine or physical therapy program for your athletes/patients, it needs to utilize Symmetry. Symmetry's Postural Alignment Technology™ protects the body from the inside out and preserves the longevity of a person's physical abilities. Every person interested in taking care of their body needs to invest in a routine. You need to take care of your body and it will take care of you – it works if you work it!

I think the world of Patrick—he is my brother from another mother— he's on this planet to help people, serve people, and make a difference in this world. Patrick means the world to me because he has done an incredible amount for me: without him, Symmetry would not have been created, and it is his creation of Symmetry that has given me the light to progress further in life. I know what it did for me and I am confident that it can change someone else's life the way it has mine.

My goal is to be able to reach one soul at a time, one body at a time, just by letting people know what Symmetry can do for them and what Symmetry did for me. If I can make someone else feel good, then I feel like I'm doing what I am here on this planet to do. I'm here to help people get a routine that I know will do a body good. Symmetry is an incredible program that will help anyone pinpoint the areas in which they have problems and provide them the tools necessary to address areas of concern. It has helped me immeasurably in my NFL career and my post career.

The book you are about to read will change your life; whether you are a practitioner who wants to enhance your practice, or someone in need of a solution to your chronic pain. It's a beautiful combination of Patrick's personal journey in creating Symmetry, to the technical understanding of how Symmetry actually works. My greatest inspiration is that, through careful study of the following pages, you will find yourself empowered with the knowledge that you, with Patrick's guidance and direction, are capable of alleviating pain and maximizing your body's health through the gift of Postural Alignment Technology.

Chapter 1

Reliance

It was the top of the 9th, 2 outs, the last game of the year, the last play of my career. We were playing the Rainbow Warriors of Hawaii and we desperately wanted to win our last game in what culminated in the strangest season I have ever experienced. The batter hit a ground ball up the middle and as I chased it into center field, I planted my left foot to make the play only to have my ankle give way, again--and just like that my career was over.

I had earned a scholarship to San Diego State University (SDSU), a division 1 NCAA school; having come from a town of only 1000 people, that was a fairly big deal. I had always wanted to play on a division-one team and through hard work and determination I had achieved that goal. Baseball to me was my first priority and college was just the avenue by which I could obtain that goal. The irony was that my chronic injuries brought me knowledge that I wasn't exactly searching for: a full understanding of the limitations and ineffectiveness of our healthcare system. I chose SDSU for two reasons; 1) It didn't snow there, and 2) it was the only college that offered me a scholarship that had anything related to Physical Therapy, the career I once thought I wanted to pursue when my baseball career was over. I knew that I wanted to be in a field where I could help people in some way, but no colleges with Physical Therapy and baseball ever recruited me. So, when It came down to choosing from the four schools that did offer me scholarships, I chose SDSU because at that time their Athletic Training program was #2 in the nation and offered a natural stepping stone to Physical Therapy school once I graduated. What I didn't anticipate was that choosing the combination of Athletic Training and baseball would change my life forever.

I entered my senior year still carrying the dream of becoming a professional major leaguer. I grew up listening to Vin Scully on the radio, spending every opportunity I could listening to the Dodgers over the waves, envisioning myself as Steve Sax turning double plays or leading off in game 1 of the World Series. It was the one thing I was really passionate about as a boy, and then a young man, and I was so close to making it a reality. So, it was natural for me to take the summer and fall going into my final season more seriously than ever before, preparing myself mentally and physically beyond anything I had done in the past. I thought I had the inside track to becoming more physically fit and knowledgeable than I had ever been by being in the Athletic Training program. I lived in the weight room and studied harder than I had ever before. I went from bench pressing 200 pounds at the end of my junior year, to 300 pounds at the beginning of my senior year. I also earned the Western Athletic Scholar Athlete of the Year award that year. However, I was also chronically injured, worse than ever before, and no one could help me. It was an incredibly frustrating experience to train day and night, seeing every practitioner I could from physical therapists to chiropractors to the team physician. I was stretched, pulled, kneaded, taped, injected, iced and adjusted, only to get temporary relief at best. This wasn't supposed to happen. I was in a field that was supposed to provide the answers for injury and pain, but no one could give me the answers I was looking for to heal my pain. Chronic ankle sprains, foot pain, left hamstring pulls, right Sacral Iliac pain, knee and shoulder pain. It was a season of cyclic annoyances that ultimately lead me to question the choice of career I had been pursuing.

After I had sprained my ankle in that last game, I was devastated. Despite all my injuries, my determination to play kept me off the bench until that last game, and I was voted Most Valuable Player for our team and All Western Player in the Western Athletic Conference. I was even invited to try out with the St. Louis Cardinals who came to our campus a week later to give us a shot at the next level. Sadly, I couldn't walk, let alone run or pivot. During the week prior to the tryout, I rehabbed my ankle just as I had so many times before, but on the day of the tryout I showed up to the training room to get taped, and it was locked. Being the end of May, the semester was over and therefore no need to keep the training room open. I stared through the window in front of the training room for about 30 minutes, hoping someone would show up to tape me. This was where I had my first revelation. I realized for the first time how dependent I was on practitioners "fixing" me when I had an injury, and the moment when I needed one the most, I found myself alone and helpless--and I panicked.

The St. Louis Cardinals. My sister had bought me one of those miniature St. Louis Cardinals' bats 15 years prior when she went on a trip to Missouri; I was sure that by holding onto that bat all those years I'd secured my fate, and now I'd been invited to try out for them. However, I found myself hopeless on the most important day of my life up to that point, all the years of hard work and determination were seemingly for naught. This was not how my career was supposed to end, in fact, I never really planned for it to end. Nonetheless, I knew that on that particular day, due to our team's disastrous record of 22 wins and 44 losses that season, not many scouts had showed up to observe our players and this would probably be my one shot to make it to the next level. Yet, here I stood, helpless and feeling sorry for myself, and ready to give up. Somehow, I pulled myself together, went home to my apartment, and taped my own ankle.

Chapter 2

Posture and Pain

There are no coincidences in life, in my opinion. After realizing that my career path needed to change, one day while running on the beach I literally ran into a former classmate of mine. She was a great friend who I often studied and hung out with, and after apologizing for running into her, I explained why I was in such deep thought, unaware that she was in my path. After listening to my woes about not knowing what career to choose, she smiled and excitedly told me the clinic she worked for was looking to hire, and what they specialized in was not taught in school, nor were they looking for anyone with great experience. I immediately went home, called the clinic, applied and was offered a position the following week! In one instant my life had changed. It felt good to have direction again.

The interview process was a bit backwards. Typically, I would be meeting first with the head of the Athletic Program, Harland Svare, the former New York Giant; then I was to meet with the director of therapy, and after that, the founder of the Egoscue method itself, Pete Egoscue. However, I met first with Pete Egoscue, because the director and Harland were away on business. Pete is a very large barrel-chested man with the bedside manner of a retired marine (which, coincidentally enough, he is). When I met with him he was silent at first—intimidatingly so—while observing me walk in. I shook his hand and walked to his office.

Once inside, Pete began by asking me if I had ever heard of him or his clinic before, and I explained that I hadn't. He then asked me why I applied for this job. I proceeded to fill him in on my past and explained my disappointment in the western medical model. I told him that I was looking for a program that I could believe in and that could possibly help me with my injuries. He laughed and said, "If you end up working here, and with what you will be learning, you really should be paying us!" I didn't know how to take that as I had no idea what he had created, but he started to explain. What he explained blew me away.

Upon observing me and knowing I had played baseball, Pete told me exactly how I stood in the batter's box, where I tended to hit the ball and where I more than likely had my pain. He was spot on. I was really impressed—as was he—but I gave him latitude as no one had ever assessed me in a way that did not involve x-rays and stethoscopes. I finally knew I had found my calling.

For the next two weeks I dedicated my time to studying the roughly 300 stretches and isometric strengthening positions—some I had learned in college, others were offshoots of yoga poses, and some I had never seen before. After that, my training consisted of observing the therapists, asking as many questions as I could, trying to figure out how this method actually worked. Two months later, I showed up to work one day and they had overbooked their clients. Thus, began my career as a Postural Therapist. I had no idea what I was doing.

There was no test for me to take, no observation of me proving I knew what I was doing: there were no manuals for me to reference; there were no steps for me to follow in creating a "menu" for my clients. However, I knew the philosophy was sound. If you have poor posture, then you are compromising your joints when you move, which can cause pain. The problem I had was that the entire method was based on viewing a person's posture and watching them walk. This is extremely subjective and hard to prove from session to session what changes have been made, especially if the client was not getting out of pain. The clients did eventually get better going through the program, but only after a great cost.

Not only was this method financially steep, but the time it took to go through the sequence of exercises was on average 60 minutes per attempt. The reason being, that there was no quantification of the method. Clients had to strip down to their underwear in order for us to observe their asymmetries, and then we would take their pictures (as if the former wasn't uncomfortable enough). Our only reference point for the success of the program was the pain itself—no different than any other therapy I had experienced. Even the most committed client would eventually stop doing their routine because of the length. Unfortunately, and since our ability to create routines was so subjective, we would end up giving too many exercises just hoping that something would stick.

I knew I was in the right field, but I also knew I was running out of passion working at this clinic. The reason I pressed on is because the method worked for me when everything else hadn't. Two years later I realized it was time to go on my own and attempt to truly figure out how this "method" worked.

I remember the exact day I made the decision to leave. I was working with a client who I had never seen before, but was still experiencing a lot of pain after five sessions, and I had no idea what to do with her. I elicited the help of the director. He came out, firmly gazed at my client as she walked up and down the hall, suggested a series of stretches, and walked away. I went to my office to digest his list and began pulling my hair out as I had no clue why he sequenced these particular exercises in the order he had chosen. With a frustrated sigh, I decided to elicit the guidance of Pete Egoscue, who grudgingly came to my aid. Pete always stood with his arms folded and one hand caressing his chin while in deep thought. After my client walked back and forth several times, Pete turned to me and commanded his orders. I quickly receded back to my office to digest his menu of exercises.

This was where I confirmed my second revelation. The two recommended sequences of exercises for the client were nowhere close to being the same. At that moment I realized that instinct cannot be taught. This method needed consistency and standardization to fully be considered a method. The next day Symmetry was born and I have never looked back.

I formally started Symmetry in 1997 with the assumption that I knew how to run a business. I was 27 and ignorant. Coupled with starting a business I had married as well. I truly believe that if everyone knew what it took to create a successful business, and marriage, for that matter, not many businesses (or marriages) would exist. I suppose this is why for the first time in our country's history, more businesses and marriages are failing than succeeding.

I had taken what I had learned at the Egoscue Method and

simply applied it to the new business, still not really knowing what I was doing, but understanding enough to get people out of pain. I knew in my heart that this wasn't good enough. Apparently, I had sent out that message because it wasn't too soon after that I received a phone call from a man named Geoff Gluckman. Geoff had also worked for Egoscue and left to start his own company a few years previous. He asked me if I was confident in what I had learned. Of course, he knew what my answer would be and so instead I asked him what was different with his method. The conversation piqued my attention enough to sign up for his course, as I had so desperately wanted some type of education while working at the Egoscue clinic. Geoff provided me with the next revelation by reintroducing me to the planes of motion. I had studied the planes of motion in college for about a day. The planes of motion are the ways the body move around gravity and give a basis for how the body operates three-dimensionally. Geoff had put Egoscue's ideas into a concrete way of explaining how the body works around right angles: thus, providing a baseline of understanding how asymmetries are derived, and therefore how to correct them.

This, however, only went so far, as I still found myself not fully understanding the process of sequencing, even though the planes of motion concept at least gave me some indication of how to compare and compartmentalize the deviations I was seeing. I remember vividly, a heated debate by a chiropractor and Geoff at his level 3 course, where there was great confusion about why Geoff picked a certain exercise in one of his examples, and why it was a better choice for the particular deviation he was discussing. The argument went on for about 30 minutes and the chiropractor could not get

Geoff to explain his theory well enough for him to let it go, and in the end Geoff told him to just trust his explanation. Deja vu. I had heard that phrase about 50 times while working at the Egoscue clinic, and I realized at that moment that there had to be a better way to explain this system beyond Geoff's theory. It was good, but not great. I found myself still at a loss of explanations that satiated my desire to fully understand how this method worked. I began to search more.

Two weeks after I was speaking to one of my clients about my experience with Gluckman, and they mentioned a chiropractor in Newport Beach that they knew thought outside the box. I really don't know what prompted me to contact this doctor, as I had been referred to many specialists before to observe their techniques who I never ended up contacting, but the timing seemed appropriate, so I called. To this day I can't remember his name, but he was a nice older gentleman that specialized in Atlas-Orthogonal work-fine neck adjustments to clear the nerve pathways from the base of the head to the body. What impressed me the most though was all the gadgets he had in his office to show his patients how misaligned they were. He had a glass foot-plate with a camera underneath to show the pressure imbalances of the feet while standing. He had a force plate analyzer that showed how the weight was divided on both legs. But one gadget impressed me the most—a fancy level that his neighbor had made for him that measured the elevation of the pelvis. A simple bubble showed his patient how uneven their pelvis was while standing, and then how even the bubble was after making one simple adjustment to the neck. What caught my attention the most wasn't the device itself, but the reaction the patient had, once they were re-measured with the level, and how impressed they were with how the bubble leveled out and how this correlated directly to a decrease in the pain they were experiencing. His patient was giddy with enthusiasm and it was at this moment that I realized the missing link from my experiences with Egoscue and Gluckman. Neither had an objective way of measuring their outcomes, therefore no way to monitor their progress from session to session. What I took home with me the most was that what this doctor had done positively affected the patient's experience by providing them a better understanding of why they felt better. I realized that I had lacked the same experiences in college and that my only reference to the success of a treatment was whether I felt better or not. Unfortunately for me I had no long-term relief and no explanations as to why, which is the story I hear every day at my clinic.

I knew in that moment that I had to make one of these devices myself. I asked the chiropractor if his neighbor would make me one, but he no longer lived near him. I immediately went to Home Depot to try and build one myself, but failed miserably. Again, timing.

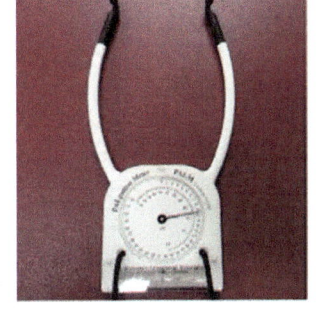

With the burning idea of figuring out how to take what Gluckman taught me and make it into an objective process, I was sitting at a warehouse in Oceanside, picking up Symmetry shirts and found a device called the Palpation Meter in a medical catalog I was glancing through. It reached out at me like one of those pop-up books I used to read as a kid. I immediately ordered one and thus began the process of Postural Alignment Technology™.

Chapter 3

Understanding Pain

If there is one thing I would like to disseminate to anyone who is suffering from chronic pain, it is simply this: understand WHY you are in pain. Take a look at these statistics on chronic pain (clinicalresearch.com):

Worldwide...

- 120 million adults (20% of the world population) suffer from pain worldwide

- 60 million—1 in 10 adults—are newly diagnosed with chronic pain each year

- 1 in 5 adults suffer from moderate to severe chronic pain

- 1 in 3 adults have trouble living independently due to pain

In the United States...

- 100 million Americans suffer from chronic pain

- 25.8 million have pain due to diabetes

- 23 million have pain due to heart disease and stroke

- 26 million between ages 20 and 64 have frequent back pain

Being in this field for 22 years now, the one thing that always makes me cringe is that the amount of chronic pain in our society each year increases. With all of the technological advancements, the newest surgeries, and the latest drugs, pain and disease becomes more and more prevalent each year. How can this possibly be with all of the brilliant minds in our medical community? To me it is simple. Prevention versus Reaction. The emphasis of treatments is completely backwards as we focus almost completely on the pain or disease itself rather than the cause of the pain or disease. Think about it: What are the treatment recommendations for chronic pain? Medication is most prevalent, followed by physical therapy, then hands-on treatments. The common denominator with all of these treatment models is a reliance on something or someone to make you "feel" better. Not one program gives you a comprehensive home plan with consistent follow-up and adjustments to make sure you are not only staying consistent with the program, but making the proper changes to allow you to maintain your progress. Most therapies certainly don't focus on preventing the issues from coming back, but rather on temporary symptom assuagement.

I was at a health fair once in San Diego, and I was speaking to the CEO of the corporation we were sponsoring. He was from Japan and we were talking about Symmetry because he was intrigued by our concept of prevention to get rid of pain. If you truly think about it, almost all disease and pain can be prevented if you are knowledgeable about what it is you are trying to prevent. However, most people don't know what they don't know, and so proceed with the mantra "if it ain't broke, don't fix it". This CEO was explaining how Eastern philosophy is all about prevention. Most Japanese corporations have their employees perform some type of yoga or stretching before they start their day. It not only helps physically, but it builds morale, thus increasing employee production. He further explained that when something critical does occur, the Japanese come to the United States because we are known for our great "reactive" medical care. Who do you think is saving the most money at the end of the day? I know this is another topic, healthcare, but if you are interested in my opinion, it doesn't matter what the healthcare system is called, but what its focus is. And trust me, it's not on getting you better.

So, is pain a good thing? No, it's great! A chiropractor once explained pain in a way I had never heard before and I have never forgotten since. He said that pain and our reaction to it is like the smoke detector in your house. What would happen if one night your alarm went off? What would you do? My first reaction would be to check for a fire. But what happens if there is no fire? This has actually happened to me. My alarm went off, I checked for a fire, which there wasn't, but the alarm kept blaring. It was 2:30 in the morning so I did what most people would do--I ripped it out of the ceiling! But what if an hour later I had awoken to a real fire? What most of us don't understand is that once you start to feel chronic pain--it doesn't matter where it is-- your body has been compensating for years to avoid it. However, before we talk comprehensively about compensation, we must first discuss what true alignment looks like and why our bodies become misaligned in the first place.

Chapter 4

True Alignment

Do you remember when you were born? Okay, how about this-- have you watched children as they grow? On average, it takes most children 12 months from the time they are born to their first step. Compared to other mammals, why does it take us so much longer to learn how to walk? Simply put, we are bipedal, or two-legged. In neuromuscular terms, it takes us longer to walk because we were designed to be vertical, and the process of being stable in a vertical position requires a very distinct learning process involving balancing to stand and then walk. We have two types of muscles in our bodies: Intrinsic and dynamic. Intrinsic muscles are the "core" muscles (no, I don't mean abs) that are designed to hold your body in a static standing position. By definition, intrinsic muscles do not change length with external force. Dynamic muscles are the "strength" muscles that are designed to move your body.

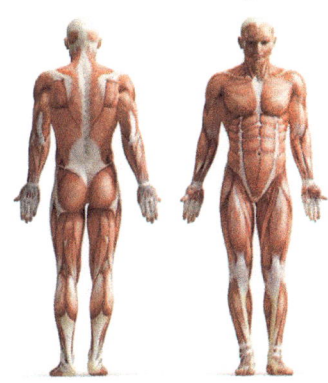

By definition, they do change length with external force. When we are learning to walk, we must go through a very specific process of educating these two groups to properly work together to efficiently and effectively hold and move our bodies. When we are first born our initial position is on our backs. Then we learn how to roll ourselves onto our stomach. Then we crawl. Then we sit. Eventually, we start to pull ourselves up to a standing position, and finally we take our first steps. This process is crucial to the proper development of our body as a whole for a plethora of reasons, which we will discuss. But none of it can be understood unless we talk about gravity.

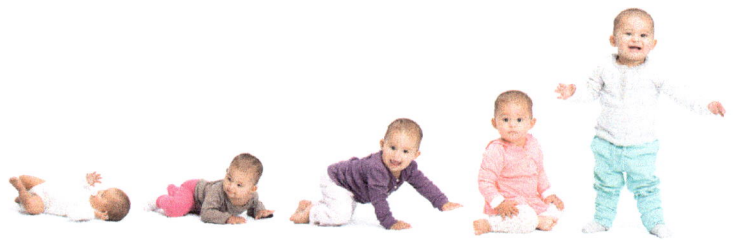

When you have seen your doctor or specialist about your chronic pain, how many of them ever used the word 'gravity' in discussing your issues? No one has ever told me that they had been discussing this with their practitioner. Why not? Because we take it for granted. Right now, you are probably sitting inside of some type of building while you are reading this book. Did you ever once consider whether the building is going to fall on you at any moment? No, because you assumed that the architects that designed it knew what they were doing. What you assumed is that the foundation is level and strong and that the walls are vertical to the foundation and supporting the ceiling which is horizontal to the floor. Every day we take things for granted, from the car we drive to the chairs we sit in, assuming they have been built correctly, but never do we consider the force they are constructed around. Understanding the laws of gravity are paramount to understanding the nature of our physical body.

If we were to assess the design the human body, how would we conclude the most efficient way for it to operate, both from a physical AND physiological perspective? First and foremost, we would know that there is a force that falls perpendicular to the earth's surface through the center of the earth. For the sake of our discussion here, it is not relevant to go deeper into the universal forces and theories, but rather that we can all agree that gravity not only exists but that it is constant. Based on this knowledge, we can take any architectural or engineering principals and apply them to our structure. Let's go back to being a child again. We discussed that it takes on average one year to get on our feet. During this process, there is a very

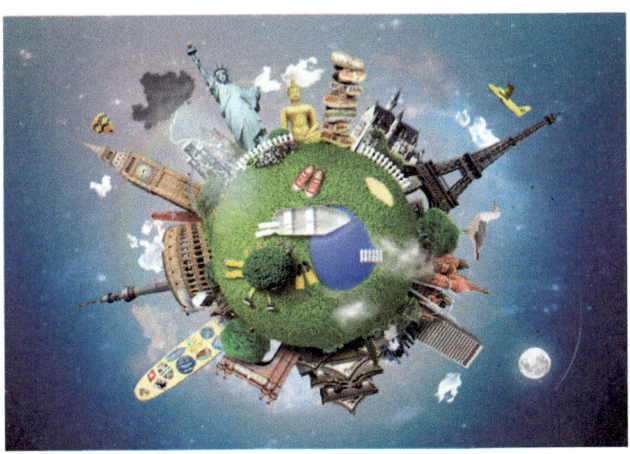

sequential pattern of development between the brain and the body. Again, for our discussion here, let's not delve into the specifics of neuromuscular makeup, but rather focus on how we would best take a human body and allow it to work the most efficiently around the downward force of gravity. Okay, so breaking it down further, we must conclude two things. One, the human body cannot exist without gravity. Two, there must be a universal design that best fits around gravity because this force IS constant. The reason it takes one year for us to learn how to walk is because movement is the most important aspect of our function and existence. The brain must coordinate the neurological development between the intrinsic and dynamic muscles around gravity in a way that best supports the entire system- in order to maximize its movement. When we are born, we do not have the neurological connection to our muscles to allow us to stand and walk immediately. Why is this so important to understand? Once again, I must emphasize that it takes us one complete year to be able to walk on two legs. This process of neurological coordination defines how our bodies were meant to be aligned, because once we learn how to move, we don't stop moving, or at least we shouldn't! Given that moving is so crucial to our existence, we must have the form to support the movement properly, thus the phrase "form follows function" was born.

Now that we have established the importance of gravity, let's take a closer look at children once they learn how to move. If you have children or have observed them, you will see that they cannot sit still. This is because the brain is created in such a way that movement feeds its growth and evolution. This is an entire topic in and of itself, but for now, let's stick to the phrase we just mentioned. If movement is priority number one, and form is the mechanism by which we allow efficient and effective movement, then we must discuss what true form is, as it relates to the necessity of movement. This is where planes of motion are vital to the overall message of this book, because it defines what true alignment is and should be.

The Planes of Motion was a topic in school that we spent about 20 minutes discussing. I not only have a patent created around these principals, but I am now developing a two-year curriculum for two universities who have asked me to bring Symmetry to its students as an optional AA degree. I currently have a three-level certification program for practitioners, empowering them to apply these principles directly within their practices. So, what are these "Planes of Motion" that are so central to my mission? We mentioned earlier about intrinsic and dynamic muscles. Intrinsic holds; dynamic moves. What this diagram shows us is not only proper alignment, but the proper starting position by which the body can move three-dimensionally

Anatomical Planes

- Anatomical position
- Anatomical planes

- Coronal (Frontal) Plane divides the body into front and back sections
- Sagittal Plane divides the body into left and right sections
  - Median - divides the body into equal left and right parts
- Axial (Horizontal or Transverse) Plane - divides the body into upper and lower segments

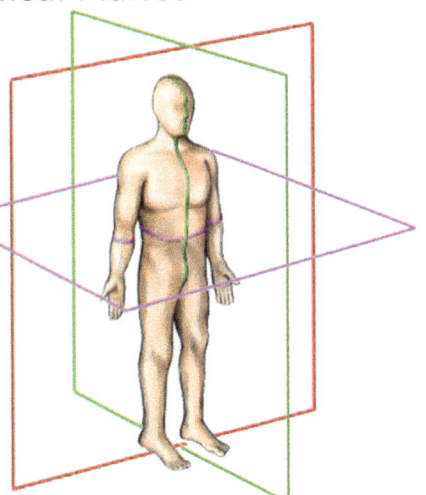

as efficiently as possible. We can either move front to back (flexion/extension), which is known as the Sagittal Plane, side to side (abduction/adduction), which is known as the Coronal Plane or the Frontal Plane, or twist (rotation), which is known as the Transverse Plane. This alignment is what children show us. From the side view (Frontal Plane) gravity should directly fall through the midline of the ear, shoulder, hip joint (greater trochanter), knee joint (lateral condyle), and ankle joint (lateral malleolus). The tilt of the pelvis from the PSIS (posterior superior iliac spine) and ASIS (anterior superior iliac spine) is the same (optimally at 10 degrees). Looking from the front view (Sagittal Plane) the spine is straight with no lateral shifts, the legs are straight (knee joints in line with the hip joint and ankle and pointing straight ahead), and the feet balanced (neither collapsed or rolled out). From the back view (Transverse Plane) the pelvis and the shoulders are level.

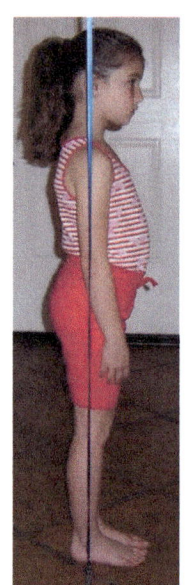

In 2004, we implemented a study at the Explorer Elementary School in San Diego to find out two things. The first was to verify my initial findings of children holding themselves according to the Planes of Motion, and the second was to find out what age-group started to show misalignment leading them away from this ideal blueprint. Our findings were astonishing; revealing the main reason why we have so much pain in our world today.

Chapter 5

Causes of Misalignment

Now that we have established that gravity does exist, and that our bodies rely on this force to exist, then movement is the key to keeping ourselves healthy and happy. However, today's environment is terrible in regard to keeping us healthy and happy, due to the fact that we stop moving at such an early age. Think about it. Has technology helped or hindered us? A few months ago, my wife and I were at a restaurant and she told me to conspicuously turn around to observe a family of five sitting at a table near us. There were three kids ranging from around 3 to 8, each one intently focused on their ASDs (anti-social devices), as my wife cleverly labels them. I'm sure they are on these ASDs at home as well, when they should be out playing in the back yard. I know when I was growing up we didn't have portable devices or Xboxes. Atari had just come out, but you had to have plenty of disposable income to afford one. I tell my kids that I remember growing up with a black and white television and we had to get up to change the channel. Today, we live in a different era due the amount of technology we are privy to and parents who are more than willing to shut their kids up and out. It's quite embarrassing to me, but this is what we have become…talking heads. Are we really surprised that our country leads the world in obesity in children? We simply do not move like my friends and I did as children. My mom had to yell at me to get inside after dark.

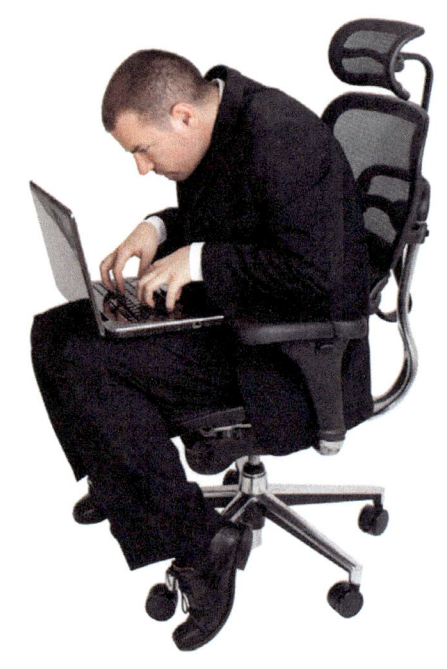

Then there is education. What age were you when you started school? On average, we all start school around five years old, and we also begin to sit. Previously I discussed the concept "form follows function". This is true for a well-functioning society where we continue to move 80% of the day our ENTIRE lives. However, because we stop moving consistently at such an early age, the intrinsic holding patterns around an extended and balanced body begin to regress, and the older we get, the more chairs we find ourselves in.

In our study at Explorer Elementary in 2004, we found that eight-year-olds already show significant misalignments. At a time when the body needs movement more than ever to support our natural design, we place kids in a desk, which impedes the natural process of keeping the body upright and extended. Therefore, sitting is THE number one reason we have chronic pain. Our intrinsic muscles are attached in a very specific, strategic way to hold our frame in its optimal orthogonal position, otherwise known as the Planes of Motion. When we sit, our frame is in its most flexed position which completely de-emphasizes the intrinsic integrity response. We were designed to be able to sit, but not for long periods of time. And the more time we sit, the less integrity our intrinsic muscles have to hold our frame. In fact, when we sit, we literally shut off two out of three planes of muscles due to the fact that we are sitting.

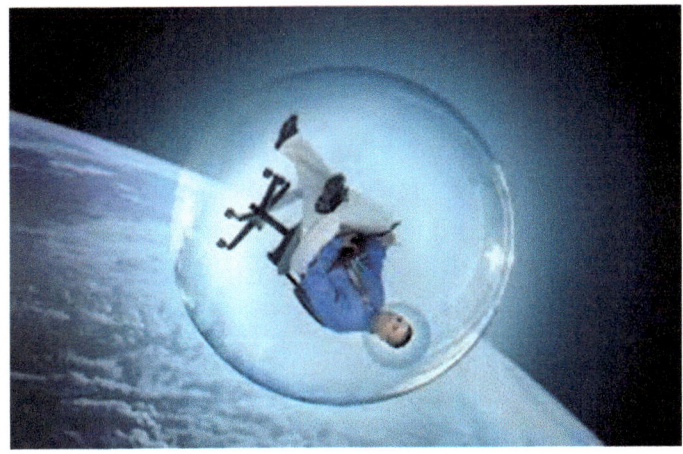

The frontal plane muscles only function when one is standing, as their responsibility is to laterally (and medially) support the body statically when standing. The transverse muscle group is also shut off because when we are sitting on our pelvis, the insertions of the rotational muscles in the pelvis have no effect on stabilizing through the torso because again, there is no extension while sitting. In her book "Sitting Kills, Moving Heals", Joan Vernikos Ph.D., the former director of NASA's Life Science Division, validated the conclusion of comparing sitting to that of being weightless in space in that it only takes up to 72 hours of non-loadbearing positioning to start negatively affecting the anti-gravitational muscles (intrinsic), thereby supporting the theory that if you don't use it, you lose it. Think about your life for a moment. You went to school at the age of 5, sat the majority of your educational life, only to graduate from college to get a job where you either sit all day long or stand in one position for long periods of time. The fact remains that even if you have a "functional" job as an adult, you already have had nearly 20 years of incorrect patterning due to not using your body as it was intended. Once you have developed that patterning, unless you are specifically intentional on correcting it, your body adds one layer at a time, one year at a time and never lets it go. Eventually your body will give up or give out and you are left with a chronic situation that you're really not sure how to reverse. At this point, the adage "form follows function" becomes reversed, because if you are standing out of alignment, then you are going to move out of alignment, which only strengthens these compensation patterns. What needs to be addressed first is the dysfunctional holding pattern of the body so that when you move, you are moving effectively and efficiently around the force of gravity. Therefore, function must follow form, otherwise you will continue to exacerbate the misalignments accrued over your lifetime and nothing will

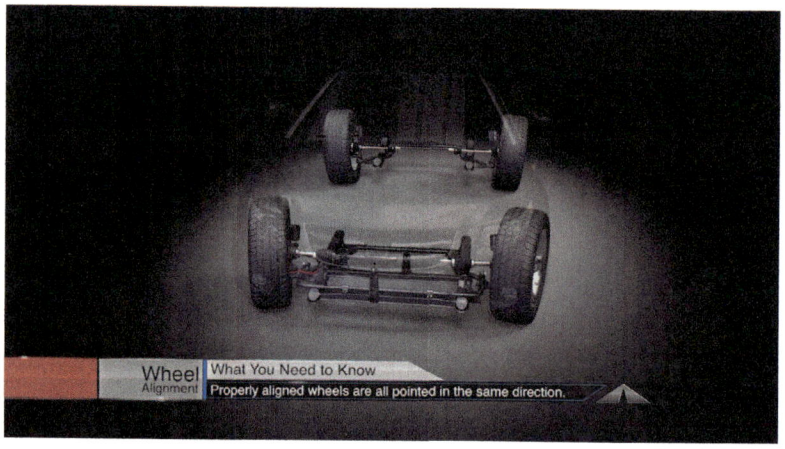

change relative to your symptoms. It would be very similar to your car being out of alignment and your tires wearing out unevenly. If you don't fix the misalignment, then new tires will wear in the same exact fashion.

The next main cause of misalignment is due to injury. I remember when I was in high school I fractured my ankle playing basketball. For six weeks, I was on crutches until my ankle healed and then I was back to my normal activities.

I was a running back in high school, getting tackled 20 times per game. I once calculated that I literally crashed on average every 5 yards nearly 500 times over my high school career. In college, I was always getting injured, the worst pain I ever felt was taking a foul ball off my tibia. When we suffer an injury, we don't think of the consequences that result from not having normal activity during the period your body recovers. Every time we put our bodies in a long-term situation of non-activity, the body must adjust, meaning we compensate. What we don't realize is that in the same way sitting causes decreased intrinsic function, so does using our body in a unilateral way for a long period of time as we recover from an injury. Six weeks is a long enough time to incorporate imbalance and misalignment in the body due to avoiding the injured site. Think about how many injuries you have sustained over your lifetime, each one adding a layer of compensation and misalignment. When we are working with a client, one thing that often happens is the reintroduction of old symptoms from a specific prior accident or injury. The reason this happens is because when we originally had the injury, we never rehabbed our body back to balance, just the area that was injured. The compensation that initiated from the injury never really leaves the body when the injured

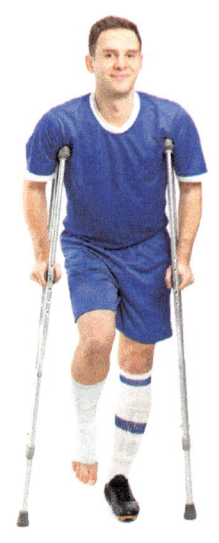

site is healed and ultimately, chronic pain is the result of our history of injuries and compensations. In my case, my injuries were consistent, at least the ones that were non-contact. I always sprained my left ankle, right quad and left hamstring; my right SI (sacroiliac) joint would always "go out", and I had chronic plantar fasciitis in both feet. Whenever I would get an injury I would go to the training room already knowing exactly what the treatment protocol would be. What bothered me the most with respect to the recurring injuries I would sustain, was the consistent lack of understanding about what I could do to prevent these injuries from happening again and again. In retrospect, I realize that the symptom was being treated and not the cause. So even though the injury would eventually heal, I was taking the same misaligned body back onto the playing field.

Repetitive stress is the next reason for misalignment. Let's recap our discussion thus far. It takes you at least one year to get to the point of walking from the time you are born. We then spend the next three years playing- jumping, twisting and running. Never sitting still. Then we get to pre-K and then kindergarten, and we take the majority of movement out of our lives. Then comes grade school, high school, and college. We sit more and more the higher the educational demand. And what for? To graduate to get a job so we can sit some more, or get a job that has us in dysfunctional positions all day. But we aren't just sitting or standing. We add a computer in front of us with a mouse. Or we stand and bend over patients all day in awkward positions. Either way, we not only have the previous years of compensations to contend with, but now we enter a profession that adds to the dysfunction. We literally

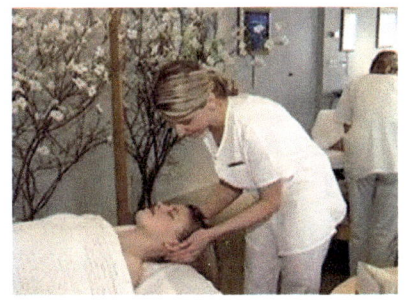

become what we do; it is the alignment version of "we are what we eat." Daily habits create just that: habits in the body that start to imprint negative structural patterns. However, it doesn't stop there. For those of us who still want to be active, we take our misaligned bodies into our activities and don't realize that we are simply adding to the dysfunction. As I mentioned in the first chapter, when I was a senior in college prior to my last season of baseball, I lived in the weight room. I went from bench-pressing 200 pounds to 300 pounds in three months. What I didn't understand is that my misaligned body was still

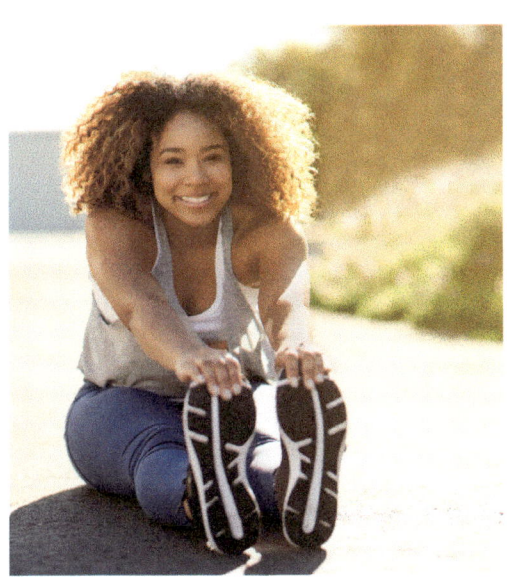

misaligned while I was lifting, and therefore all I was doing was making my dysfunctions stronger. I know for a fact that this was the lead contributor to my increased injuries that year.

Furthermore, whenever I stretched, I always felt worse. Why? Because I was stretching out the tight muscles; up until now logic dictates that stretching out tight muscles would be a natural focal point to getting out of pain, right? Wrong! Tight muscles, as we will learn shortly, are there to provide some type of stability to an imbalanced frame. We will be talking much more about compensation and how that intertwines with pain and performance, but for now, understand that your repetitive stress on an imbalanced frame is causing more and more imbalance. What this simply means is that your daily, monthly, and yearly habits continually add to your imbalanced frame unless you prepare your body for each daily routine that you put yourself into. So, stretching, for the sake of stretching, and without the combination of some type of strengthening, can result in more pain or create injury. When have you ever heard of this before?!!

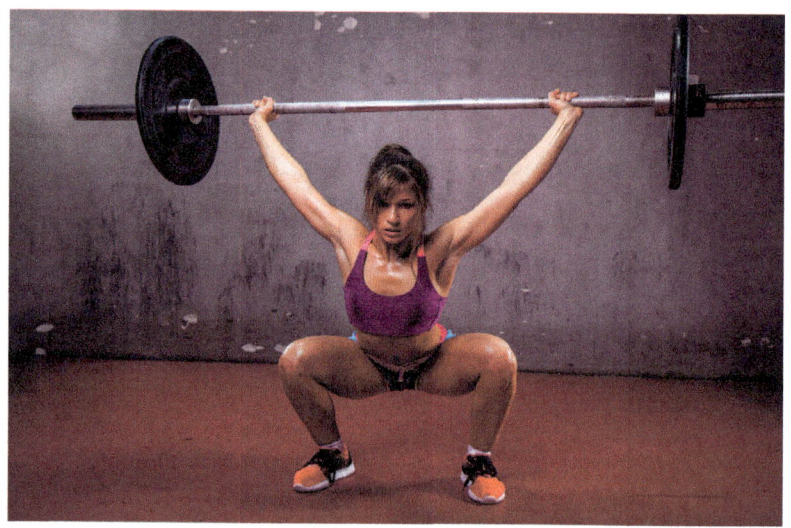

Notice the asymmetries during this lift

Sports dominance is another cause of misalignment. In the 20 years of experiencing postural dysfunctions, we have come across thousands of athletes. There is no better explanation of "you are what you do" than to take a look at sports and how it creates bad habits. In 2003 I was at the Las Vegas airport with my wife and we passed by a college team waiting to board their plane. They were all wearing their team gear but it wasn't clear exactly what type of team they were. I turned to my wife and explained to her that they were the swim team, and to my surprise she made a bet that I was wrong! So, she went up to one of the members and asked, and came back with a grimace on her face, because I was right!

In 2004 I was flown up to the University of Washington (UW) to work with Steve Emtman who was the strength and conditioning coach for UW at the time. Steve had been my very first student with Symmetry Core in 2001 and when he was given the job at UW he and I immediately talked about getting his athletes aligned. What was very interesting was when I worked with the different teams it was very apparent how their patterns were developed due to the different type of sport in which they were involved. Track and field; sprinters were very frontal-plane deviated; hurdlers were very transverse-plane deviated. Swimmers were VERY frontal-plane deviated, which is why I could tell at the Las Vegas airport that the team we saw were indeed swimmers. You see, when we look at swimmers, the first thing we must understand is that we weigh 10% of our body weight when in the pool. Spending hours in the water automatically shuts off the intrinsic muscular system as it pertains to dealing with gravity. There is no vertical load-bearing taking place while swimming, therefore the strength that occurs is almost strictly dynamic as one moves through the water. Due to this lack of vertical loadbearing, the frontal plane muscle groups are very limited in their recruitment as they mainly function in standing postures. When I observed the swim team at the airport, their sport posture was very obvious to me because when looking at their profiles, their hips and head were very forward, traps very enlarged and engaged, and lats overdeveloped as well.

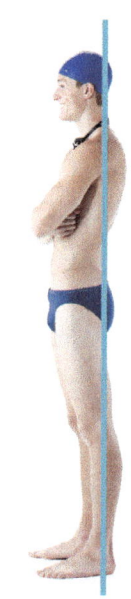

Typical Swimmer's Posture

Az Hakim was part of the "Greatest Show on Turf" when he played with the St. Louis Rams during their Super Bowl win in 1999-2000. As mentioned in the forward, I met him in 2005 when I was introduced to him by the former New York Giant and coach, Harland Svare with whom we worked with intimately in San Diego. At this point in his career, Az was picked up by the New Orleans Saints and during pre-season he suffered multiple hamstring pulls. One day Az called me and told me that the trainers with the Saints were not addressing his real issues, because all they were doing was treating his hamstring. Most of the issues most athletes develop are directly related to their strength training. If you look at the first picture of Az (next page), you will see how forward he is in the first picture. When most athletes strength-train, they work mainly in the sagittal plane, meaning that almost every movement in the weight room is linear, consisting of flexion and extension. From the bench press to the squat, athletes are disproportionately training by working primarily in one plane, which decreases the function structurally in the other two. What ends up happening is that the weaker the lateral plane becomes, the harder it is for the body to hold itself upright and aligned in this plane. As the body becomes weaker in the frontal plane and stronger in the sagittal plane, the more forward the hips move, thus prompting a response from the hamstrings in order to keep the body from falling over. Hence the true issue is weakness in the frontal plane which provokes a compensatory tightness in the hamstring, which is in the sagittal plane. When an athlete proceeds with treatment only around pain, such as the hamstring in Az's case, nothing will release long term if the initial cause is not addressed.

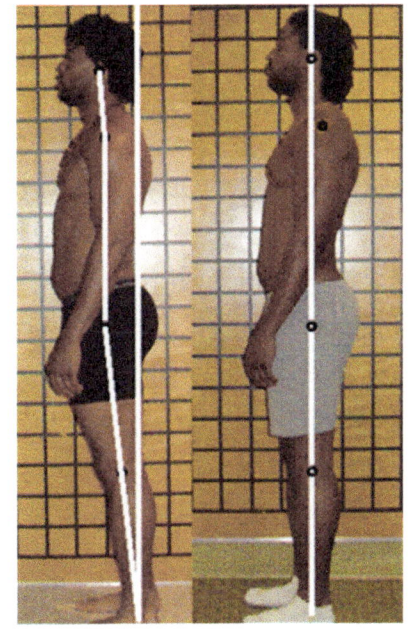

Az flew me out to the Saint's facility after pulling his hamstring for the third time, and after one postural alignment treatment, he was out running the next day, and in full gear four days later. He never had a hamstring pull again.

Genetics is the last reason for misalignment. Although this diagnosis, in my opinion, is handed out too frequently, there are cases that directly or indirectly lead to the body not being aligned. However, you must determine whether genetics truly cause misalignment or not. In some scoliotic cases, this will absolutely lead to misalignment. BUT there are two types of "scoliosis", so one must rule out which one is genetic and which one is a product of your environment. Many times, I get clients in that say they have been diagnosed with a leg length discrepancy. I am here to tell you that this is just not as prevalent as you might think. The only true way you can determine if one has a leg length discrepancy, is through x-rays, and then measuring the length of each individual leg bones. However, even with that accomplished, you are still not considering joint compression and compensation in all planes that may affect the overall loadbearing instability. One cannot lay a patient on a table, wiggle the legs a few times, and show you a picture of one foot further than the other to properly determine whether one leg is longer than the other.

In any case, don't let a diagnosis of genetics set you in a space of blind acceptance to explain your chronic pain. Even if you can verify that there is a genetic component to your misalignment, you still have all the prior four reasons that add to this dysfunctional pattern, which still need to be addressed and corrected. Using me as an example, I believe that genetics played a large part of my problems. Just look at this picture of me when I was five years old. No doubt that the body I was given was genetically manipulated. However, I blame it on being the youngest of six kids and getting the remains of the gene pool (my dad's name is actually Gene!). I always knew growing up that I wasn't put together all that well, and that it somehow had to relate to the pains from which I suffered. No one else ever did, but I knew. But, it didn't matter once I found the solution.

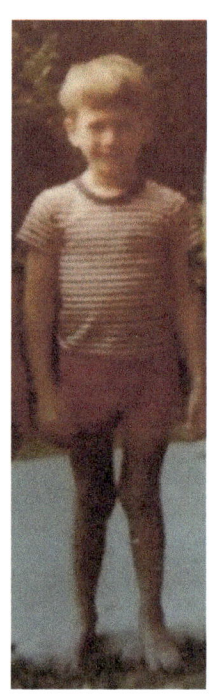

Chapter 6

The Physics of Posture -

Newton's Third Law

Symmetry can be defined simply as dealing with gravity and the laws of the universe. Whenever we get a client in front of us, we ask them if anyone has ever explained their pain as it relates to gravity. The answer inevitably is 'no'. This is because we tend to move pain to the forefront of the perceived problem and therefore the majority of the conversation is focused on the pain itself. For example, many of our clients are very excited to show us their X-rays or MRI reports. They assume we will also want to talk about these reports because that is what they are used to talking about when dealing with their pain. To us, the pain is simply the by-product of systemic breakdown due to years of dysfunction and not a complete reason in and of itself. Newton's third law states that "For Every Action There is an Equal and Opposite Reaction". This law is the basis from which Symmetry was created and it remains the most important aspect because we can always depend on gravity. Gravity is defined as the force of attraction by which terrestrial bodies tend to fall toward the center of the earth. In Physics terms this means that gravity is a constant, or "K". Just

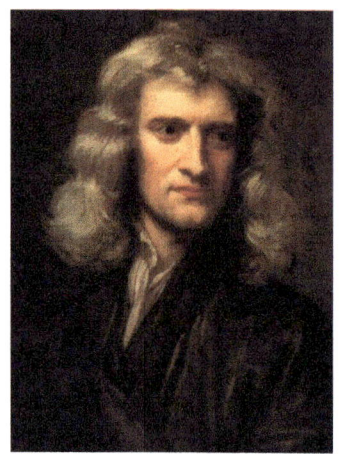 as an architect designs a building, or an engineer, a car, the number one issue they focus on is gravity and the forces that apply to the structures surrounding it, whether static or dynamic. Newton's Laws all pertain to this, but his third law in particular specifically addresses postural deviations because we are focusing on static holding patterns, and thereby on intrinsic muscles. This constant that we can count on is twofold: 1) gravity falls perpendicular to the surface of earth; 2) any structure must react directly in opposition to that force in order to hold itself upright and move effectively and efficiently. When we do not apply the reaction to the force of gravity in a constant and equal way, then ANY structure will be forced to adjust. This is the definition of compensation.

Compensation is the intent to improve any defect by the excessive development or action of another structure or organ of the same structure (Wikipedia). Given the force of gravity, if the foundation of a building is not level or strong enough, then it can be assumed that the walls will be under stress due to this imbalance. When we look at any structure, there is a fundamental understanding of balance that we instinctively take for granted. You assume that your car is aligned properly. You assume that the building you are in now was constructed correctly and that the walls will not fall down on you. What we also assume and know instinctively is that if these structures are not aligned, then there will be a compensation that will occur, such as a tire that wears unevenly as I previously mentioned. If we were to initially assume that the issue is <u>not</u> with the alignment and solely with the tire, at some point we would question why each new replaced tire is wearing in the exact same way as its predecessor. When we are discussing compensation with regards to our frame, we take the approach in most cases that the pain is not associated with the alignment of the body, or in this case, the misalignment. However, we must understand the nature of compensation and why it occurs in the first place and then relate it to the pain that we feel. Here are two main reasons:

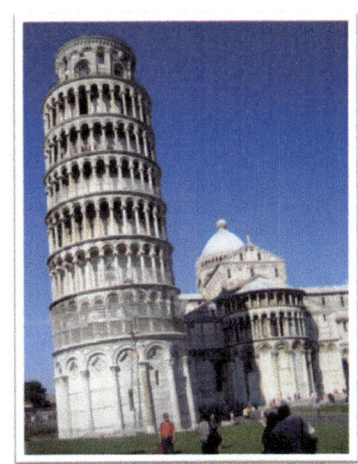

Reason #1. The main reason that the body will compensate is because our sympathetic nervous system is such that pain will be avoided at all costs if the brain detects a weakness or imbalance in our system. Its general action is to mobilize the body's nervous system fight or flight response (Wikipedia), which is a physiological reaction that occurs in response to a perceived harmful event or attack, or threat to survival. The body constantly aims to maintain homeostasis, which is derived from the Greek, *homeo* or "constant" and *stasis* or "stable", and means remaining stable or remaining the same. The human body manages a multitude of highly complex interactions to maintain balance or return systems to functioning within a normal range. These interactions within the body facilitate compensatory changes supportive of physical and psychological functioning. This process is essential to the survival of the person and to our species.

Reason #2. The second reason our bodies compensate is

due to the righting reflex: "The righting reflex, also known as the Labyrinthine righting reflex, is a reflex that corrects the orientation of the body when it is taken out of its normal upright position. It is initiated by the vestibular system, which detects that the body is not erect and causes the head to move back into position as the rest of the body follows. The perception of head movement involves the body sensing linear acceleration or the force of gravity through the otoliths, a structure in the saccule of the inner ear and angular acceleration through the semicircular canals. The reflex uses a combination of visual system inputs, vestibular inputs, and somatosensory inputs to make postural adjustments when the body becomes displaced from its normal vertical position. These inputs are used to create what is called an efference copy. This means that the brain makes comparisons in the cerebellum between expected posture and perceived posture, and corrects for the difference." (Wikipedia)

The righting reflex is one of the biggest examples of compensation and gravity due to the fact that your eyes must always be level with the horizon in order to maintain balance and equilibrium. What we haven't taken into account however is the fact that once your body becomes structurally misaligned, we spend a lifetime utilizing this reflex to literally keep our heads on straight. The question isn't whether the head has to be balanced, but what triggers the righting reflex in the first place. This, again, is where Newton's third law comes into effect because the righting reflex is nothing more than Newton's third law in action, because for every compensation there is an equal and opposite physical compensation.

Check out this picture and ask yourself what is the first thing that pops out at you. At first glance you probably will notice how uneven this person's shoulders are as designated by the stripes on her shirt. However, if you look more closely, you will see that her pelvis is also uneven. This is where we must break the body down into its basic parts and explain it in terms of physics. What we must assess is what came first, the chicken or the egg? Did the elevated shoulder come first, or the elevated hip?

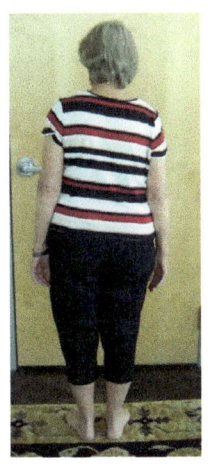

When a client comes into our office, we don't look at them in terms of pain as we have already discussed, but rather as a delicate system of levers and pulleys. Leverage is defined as the mechanical advantage or power gained by using a lever. A lever is defined as a rigid bar resting on a pivot, used to help move a heavy or firmly fixed load with one end when pressure is applied to the other; i.e., bones. A pulley is defined as a device for overcoming resistance at one point by applying force at some other point; i.e., muscles. Why is this necessary to understand? First, the body works best when it is as extended and balanced as possible in three-dimensional space. We again define this as the planes of motion. If the body is in its correct orthogonal position, then all the bones (levers) and all the muscles (pulleys) will be in what we call harmonic tension, which simply means that in the static standing position, all the muscles, both intrinsic and dynamic, are at their proper length, and therefore leveraged to hold and move the body in its most efficient way possible. Plato, in his Theory of Forms, states that "Beauty of form is that which moves with the least amount of energy."

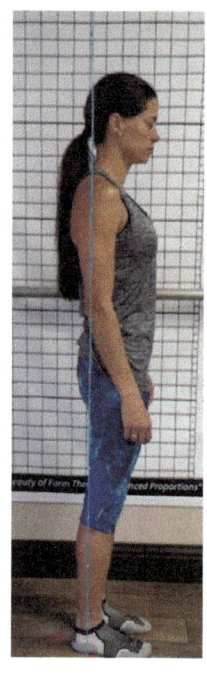

Taking into consideration levers/bones and pulleys/muscles when we are assessing the body, we must break the body down further into two simple parts- the foundation or motor unit (also known as the locomotor unit) which is comprised of the pelvis and legs, and the passenger unit, which is comprised of the upper torso. It is important to label the body using these two physics terms because we must begin to understand where leverage is originated in the body and how it relates to pain and gravity. The pelvis in our research is the most important part of the body because this is where the line of gravity should bisect the body. It is further defined by the center of mass (COM), which is the unique point where the weighted relative position of the distributed mass sums to zero. The distribution of mass is balanced around the center of mass and the average of the weighted position coordinates of the distributed mass defines its coordinates. So, how do WE define COM? Again, simply by the Planes of Motion. If you take the Transverse, Frontal and Sagittal planes and assess where they intersect, this represents the COM, and theoretically, if you are completely aligned along all three planes, then the COM should be located at the second or third sacral joint, or just superior of the acetabulum (hip joint). In most studies of the COM of the human body, the results are located much higher than this, usually in the lumbar or in some studies, the lower thoracic region. The reason for this is because we spend the majority of our lives sitting, and what we had mentioned previously is that when we sit we completely disengage the frontal plane muscle group because there is no response for stability of these muscles while sitting. Then, when one does stand, due to the inactivity and weakness of these muscles, the pelvis is thrust forward due to lack of lateral stabilization, and thus the COM is forced upwards initiating a complete different weighted relative position of the distributed mass. The upper body, or the passenger unit, is then forced to rebalance back in order to sustain the righting reflex, which can be further defined as not only rebalancing the head, but rebalancing the head back over the pelvis - this is the true aspect of how equilibrium works. In other words, your brain not only has to have the head level through the use of sight, but also cannot ultimately stabilize itself without proprioceptively balancing itself over the pelvis, as the brain instinctively knows that in order to move anywhere, this relationship must be intact. So, as the pelvis is thrust forward in the above analogy, and the torso is rebalanced back, the head must then reposition back over

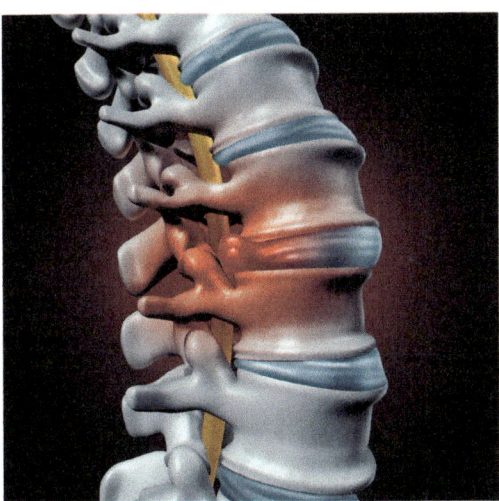

the pelvis, which is the basic posture you see with people who sit for a career. What is then caught in the middle of this balancing act? The spine; and this is not what the spine was intended to do, which is to support the entire body. This is the main reason the majority of people in the world suffer from lower back pain.

Now, taking into consideration that the motor unit is responsible for carrying the passenger unit, and that the COM is very critical, let's talk about kids again. The reason almost all children up to the age of nine have a 10-degree pelvic tilt is because from a leverage standpoint, it creates the most optimal holding position for all joints three-dimensionally. The 10-degree tilt supports the dynamic tension that I just explained and allows for the spine to be positioned optimally as well. If you look at the lateral view of the spine, it is composed in such a way to perform two main functions: 1) to provide protection for the nervous system, and 2) to provide support for the passenger unit. If the tilt of the pelvis is more than 10 degrees, then the lower spine and above becomes too extended. If the tilt of the pelvis is less than 10 degrees, then the lower spine and above becomes too flexed. Either way it leads to compression, which is directly related to almost ALL diagnoses given regarding the back. If you suffer from pain in ANY joint, you can be assured that you are compressed in that joint or joints.

Let's check back in with our subject again and go back to the question of the chicken or the egg. Symmetry determines that the COM is compromised because we are not using our foundation the way it was intended. Therefore, what begins to break down first is the integrity and balance of the motor unit due to our environmental "miscues" and lack of consistent movement from an early age that is required to keep the homeostasis between the motor unit and the passenger unit. Again, the adage of "form follows function" was true in the early years, but because we lose function at an early age, form also begins to lose function as well. If we simply take a subject and try to start moving it more, the form still stays dysfunctional and therefore tends to exacerbate the structural compensations with movement. Looking at the woman in the striped shirt, we determined that her compensations began mainly with the imbalance of the pelvis or motor unit in the transverse plane, which causes the reaction of the righting reflex; this is the case for most clients. In her case, the elevation of the left hip caused an offset of the lumbar spine towards the elevated hip, which caused the reaction of her left shoulder to elevate to reposition her head. When assessing one's posture, ultimately, we must determine which plane we must address **first** in order to correct years of accrued dysfunction. This is why we were awarded a patent: Symmetry creates a personalized and evolving sequence of the isometric stretches and strengthening positions that are derived from 21 specific measurements taken at each visit. The before and after pictures you see here are from the first session. Her issues were two bulged discs in her neck, with radiating pain down her arm, and her doctor wanted to perform surgery. However, since Symmetry doesn't focus solely on pain, we went after the cause. You can see that in the "after" picture, her shoulders are much more level, even though we did not directly address the upper body. She came in with a level of 8 on the pain scale, and left with a level of 2 and never had the surgery her doctor recommended. She couldn't understand why we didn't treat her neck like everyone had done previously, but when she was through with her routine, she didn't care. It worked and now she had access to a long-term solution with the tools and support we provided for her.

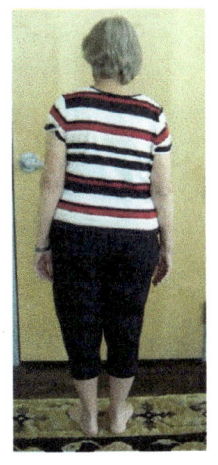 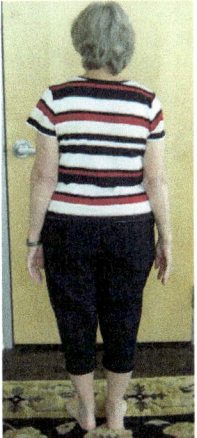

Here is another case to look at. The picture you see here is of a client (Jim) who came in 4 months after a hip-replacement. He was still in pain and walking with a limp. I showed him this Frontal Plane view and asked him what was wrong with this picture. In his beautiful British accent, he said, "I never realized my head was that bloody forward!" To this day, I'm still amazed by the surprised reactions clients have to their photos, given that other treatments never highlighted their misalignments.

Whenever I give a seminar to practitioners, I always ask who in the room takes pictures of their clients, whether for the first session or at each session. I am lucky if I see two hands raised. The next question I ask is "Why don't you?" Mostly I get the answer, "Because we were never taught to!" I already know what the answer is going to be, because client participation is not the priority in higher education. Most of what practitioners learn is how to treat a patient or client, rather than how to teach them to treat themselves. It's the old classic Bible story about fishing;

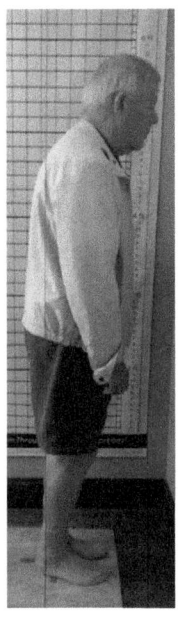

you can give a man a fish and momentarily satiate his hunger, or you can teach him to fish, which is the more sustainable solution. Generally, there is no real incentive to show people what they look like after treatment, because the common emphasis is to focus on how they feel after a treatment. Our philosophy at Symmetry is to not only show clients their postural progress from session to session, but more importantly, to measure their progress from session to session. I know I keep teasing you with hints about the process, but I really want you to read the entire book! In any case, if you have never looked at yourself in the mirror, you might want to take a closer look. Or, have someone take pictures. Later on, we will give you steps to check your own posture and see how you compare to three-dimensional alignment!

Okay, so now let's talk more about our British client. This is a 75-year-old man who had a complete left hip replacement. Looking at his profile on the previous page, you can see how forward his load-bearing joints were, from head to knee. Again, in physics terminology, we are attuning to the Center of Mass concept. We had mentioned that when properly aligned, the COM should be around S2-3 or slightly lower. When our static posture starts to deviate away from its planar stability points, then this directly effects the COM. Take a look at this picture. Just using your own subjective eye, which leg do you think he is leaning more onto? Which hip do you think was replaced? If you answered, "left hip", then you would be correct! When you add his profile picture along with this posterior view, you will determine that the way the body must hold itself up due to his compensation pattern is mainly through his left side and lower than normal COM, in other words, his left hip. You see, when we compensate over a lifetime, our body tends to wear out at the point of the COM adjustment, or where the body has reacted the most to these compensations to help balance out the body. As I mentioned previously, this is why most people suffer from lower back issues; because the back is doing way more work than it was designed to perform. In this case, Jim compensated in a way that forced him to use his left hip more than it was intended. However, the left hip is the victim of his compensation pattern, not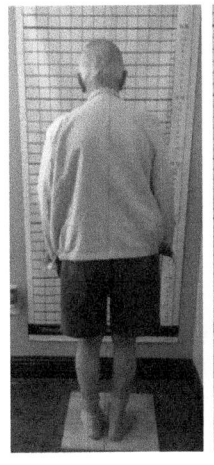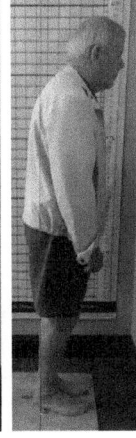

the cause. Once Jim got his left hip replaced, you can see in these pictures that the same misaligned frame still existed. Therefore, the same compensation patterns were still occurring, and he still landed more heavily on his left hip, which is why he still had pain! My biggest argument with surgery is NOT related to the surgery itself, but the lack of patient preparation prior to surgery. We call it "prehab". You see, the majority of surgeons are trained in surgery, not physics. When they show you the MRI or X-ray, and tell you that the reason you have pain is clearly diagnosed, they fail to tell you that your entire

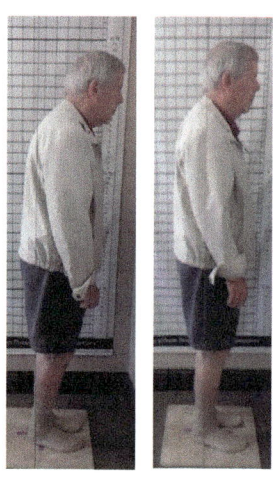

body has completely compensated. It is this compensation which has led to your specific "problem", which is actually a "reaction" to the initial harm or threat to your system as a whole. Perhaps you have the procedure done, and a day or week later you feel better because the pressure on the nerve was relieved, but your tires are still going to wear out because your frame is still off. When we get clients in to see us who are on track for surgery, our first intent is to prevent

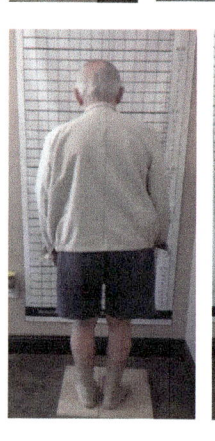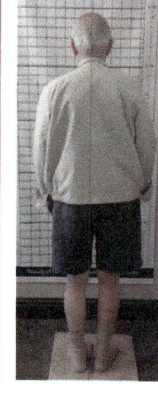

the surgery, and we have succeeded many times. However, even if the surgery cannot be avoided, the body needs to be "fixed" prior to the surgery so that the recovery is easier and more importantly, to avoid future surgeries! Again, we call this "prehab". Check out Jim's first-session pictures, after just 20 minutes of the AlignSmart™ exercises that Symmetry draws from. The real interesting thing about this first routine is that I kept Jim on the floor in a supine position throughout the entire sequence. One of the factors we use to determine the proper sequencing of a corrective exercise routine is called "ramping". It is equivalent to what I previously discussed about the development process from birth to standing, and how our individual process mimics this patterning. Sometimes I get clients who are just too compensated and cannot get off the floor due to the complexity of their dysfunctions. I don't mean that they literally can't get off the floor; in Jim's case, he clearly walked into our clinic on his first visit, and walked out of our clinic when he was through with his visit. What I mean is if I had taken him off of the floor during his initial corrective sequence, the entire connection would have been lost because his patterning was too engrained. Remember the levers and pulleys? If you try and rebuild the structure too fast, it will always default to its defensive point, or the state that feels the safest, even if that state is dysfunctional. Jim left much more aligned even though I didn't take him off of the floor during his treatment routine.

In the following chapters, I am going to lay out a more comprehensive technical explanation of physics, gravity, compensation and its effects on our structure, which I have only hinted at in the previous chapters. These chapters set the stage for a more in-depth explanation of how Symmetry's AlignSmart™ system actually works and why I was awarded a patent for this technology.

Chapter 7

Benefits of Structural Alignment

Structural alignment is important because we live on the planet earth, which is subject to the constant downward force of gravity, as we have discussed. In order to balance erect on two limbs on earth's surface we must: A) Counter the downward forces and B) Do so in the most efficient manner possible. The primary focus of our existence should not be battling gravity. Yet without realizing it, this is what the majority of us are spending our energy on. Symmetry's Postural Alignment Technology™ Program is designed to reinstate our structural integrity, thereby freeing up our energy for other types of activities and functions that help develop our lives so we can progress as a species.

A. Importance of structural alignment

The erect posture is an end result of a very dynamic process of checks and balances. It is what is achieved when the various systems of the body including the skeletal, muscular, and nervous systems, are in balance with each other and the external environment. However, this is not a static state. Therefore, our ability to stand erect is a continual process of adaptation to both internal and external stimuli.

Structural alignment is defined as skeletal correctness in the human body. It is essentially what is achieved when the skeletal frame is positioned perpendicular to the earth's surface and the force of gravity. This right angle (ninety degree) relationship between our body and the environment forms the criterion for both anatomical and physiological correctness, as well as psychological and emotional well-being. When this right-angle fundamental is achieved, the skeletal system as a whole operates at its highest level, achieving the most amount of work with the least amount of effort. As we've established, anatomical correctness is when the three planes of the body divide the body equally to form right angles at all eight load bearing joints. This will position the body perpendicular to the earth's surface, which will enable the skeleton to carry the majority of the body's weight with minimal muscular tension.

Physiological correctness is when the organ systems of the body operate effectively and efficiently. In other words, the organs are spaced sufficiently apart to: A) receive adequate nutrition (water, oxygen, minerals and vitamins) from the circulatory system and B) expand and contract maximally. This can only be achieved if the body is in a state of anatomical correctness. The inter-relatedness of physiological and anatomical correctness can be readily observed in the following example: The effect of posture on the heart. One of the axial skeletons purposes is to house and protect our organ system. Every organ is packed into this bony casing like a jigsaw puzzle, with every piece fitting perfectly against the next. There is no room for anything else. Organ walls consist of a labyrinth of veins and arteries that carry nourishment to, and waste away from their cells. Any skeletal misalignment leads to compensation. Compensation, in this context, means that the space that these organs fit into is changing. Should the change be one of decreased space (as in the prevalent rounded shoulder posture/kyphosis) the result will be organ crowding. Organ crowding inhibits the ability of the lungs to expand fully and take in enough oxygen. It cannot, therefore, provide adequate oxygen to the rest of the organ systems, which include the heart. If the heart is undernourished, it will be weak and unable to pump enough blood to the brain and the body. Without adequate oxygen and nutrients carried in the blood the various organ systems will soon become undernourished and weak, and their tissue will begin to atrophy and die. Cardiovascular Disease (CVD) results from a combination of factors, but all are aspects of organ crowding and inability to perform their intended job description.

In summary, when the bones are not perpendicular to the earth's surface and the line of gravity, an optimal internal environment, where the organ systems of the body can operate 100% effectively and efficiently, cannot be maintained. Nor can the skeleton carry the majority of the body's weight with minimal muscular tension. What this means is that our body will hold excess tension in and around its load bearing joints, leaving the organ systems weak and undernourished. These compromised physical states severely inhibit our ability to live our lives completely; the fundamental inhibiting factor being fatigue and subsequent weakness.

Our corporeal energy system is a closed system. What this means is that we have a limited amount of internally-derived energy, and only so much more that can be created from external sources such as food. In the human body, all things are not considered equal. Therefore, functions of more importance for survival, such as our heart pumping, will be given higher priority and afforded more energy if required. For example: Mr. Joe is having a heart attack. All his available energy will be directed towards coping with the sudden change in status quo and in the reestablishment of homeostasis. It doesn't matter how long ago he ate or what deadlines at work he was thinking about; he will not feel hungry nor will he continue to think about work. His body has a new priority; that of getting enough blood pumped out of his heart to his brain. The same would be true if Mr. Joe's posture resembled that of the letter "C" (kyphotic posture). This posture demonstrates an anterior/posterior imbalance, which can also be called frontal plane deviation; it results in the inability of the body to maintain its right angle fundamental and remain perpendicular to the earth's surface, most efficient position for the human body to be in. What this means is that Mr. Joe should be able to walk, sit, and think with minimal muscular effort. However, this is not the situation. A lot of Mr. Joe's energy will go to his muscular and skeletal systems as they attempt to reestablish their anterior/posterior homeostasis. Over time, if Mr. Joe does not do anything to improve his situation and his posture remains the same, then reestablishing energy requirement will increase. Not only will it become harder to stand and move, but in addition his various other systems will become less and less efficient and eventually cease operating due to a lack of adequate nutrition and atrophy. Disorders of the digestive system and colon can be pervasive in clients with kyphosis due to organ crowding and the fact that the body perceives activities such as digestion to be less important, from a basic survival perspective, than standing erect, moving, and breathing. Roger Sperry won the Nobel Prize for physiology of medicine for his discoveries concerning the functional specialization of the cerebral hemispheres. The summary of his work is described in this quote; "Better than 90% of the brain's output is directed toward maintaining your body in its gravitational field. Therefore, the less one spends on one's posture, the more energy is available for healing, digestion and thinking."

B. Case Study: A Sprained Ankle

The affected ankle joint is unable to be utilized as a load bearing structure. Therefore, it can no longer provide for absorption and dispersion of ground reaction forces, nor can it act as the fulcrum for the foot lever, which is the mechanism by which the body propels itself forward; or walking, as it is more commonly known. This means that the affected ankle has led to the entire system being unable to perform its most fundamental and unique function, that of bipedal ambulation. This lack of functioning, both muscularly and skeletally, will affect all contingent systems such as the circulatory, endocrine, and lymph systems that rely on the equal use and distribution of gravity to perform their functions. What this demonstrates is that skeletal correctness affects us on a physical level. However, skeletal correctness also affects us emotionally and psychologically. The restoration of physical balance and function within a person provides stability in the physical realm, thereby facilitating choices of how they respond to physical, mental, emotional, and energetic challenges (Gluckman, *Muscle Balance and Function*). Today, a 60-hour workweek is commonplace, as is driving a car, traveling, going to the movies, and working out. Stop and think for a minute how you would feel if you could not sit for more than 20 minutes without experiencing excruciating pain. How would this impact your life and how would you feel about yourself and your life? Symmetry sees many clients who have not been to the movies, or traveled, or had sex in years. These clients report feeling out of control, frustrated and depressed; in addition, their bodies hold these feelings and manifest them physically. The postural evaluations I perform as part of Symmetry allow me to observe the emotional stance of the person. It is an opportunity to visually and auditorily assess the messages coming from my client.

The case study of an ankle sprain is only a minor disruption of homeostasis. Therefore, it should, if logic prevails, only lead to minor compensations within the system. However, if you have ever sprained your ankle like I have; you know there is nothing minor about it. Yet, in the scheme of possible compensation and dysfunction, a sprained ankle is still considered minor. One can, therefore, imagine the level of compensation the body must undergo, and subsequent fatigue it will suffer, in order to cope with disorders such as scoliosis, kyphosis, or spina bifida, which are disorders of the axial skeleton and, therefore, effect the system at its core structural level.

Chapter 8

The Physics of Right Angles

The goal of Postural Alignment Technology™ is to re-establish the body's balance and function in reference to the force of gravity, and to return it to its ability for movement in all planes and ranges of motion. This will return the body to being bilateral with the left side being a mirror image of the right side. From a skeletal structure perspective, this will occur when every load bearing joint, namely the ankles, knees, hips and shoulders, lies in parallel horizontal relation to each other and to the ground, in healthy relation to the plumb line of gravity; these joints should all face forward, and therefore produce three dimensional right angles. These right angles will then be able to distribute forces equally to the appropriate structures. When such bilateralism is achieved, and movement is restored, large forces, upwards of 100 times one's body weight, can be quite easily managed by the body without excessive strain, attrition, or pain.

Previously, I mentioned that the optimal pelvic tilt is 10 degrees, which is what we found in measuring hundreds of children up to the age of 9 years old. The reason this makes sense is that when you analyze the spine in its purest form, in young children, the angle of the PSIS to ASIS creates a 90-degree angle in relation to the 4th lumbar vertebra through to the 2nd sacral joint. This creates the most effective position for the lower lumbar vertebrae to support the entire spine on top of the pelvis, in terms of both shock absorption and nerve protection. Anything less than 10 degrees in the pelvic tilt will cause too much flexion in the lower lumbar spine, which will echo through the thoracic and cervical spine as well; anything more than a 10-degree tilt of the pelvis will cause too much extension in the lumbar spine, and the effects of this will also carry through to the thoracic and cervical spine. Either way, if the pelvic tilt is less or more than 10 degrees, the spine will compress on itself which ultimately leads to pain regardless of the diagnosis you are given.

It is very important to acknowledge that the real indication of true bilateralism is not so much skeletal "perfection", but the ability for the body as a whole to be supported as efficiently as possible around the force of gravity. Some experts argue that there is no such thing as true "symmetry" in the human body, but I argue that within our first five years of life, we are as close to symmetrical as possible and thereafter our negative environmental cues cause a distortion in the developmental process, related back to when we discussed causes of misalignment. Given that Postural Alignment Technology™ works to reeducate the neurological system, we must focus on neurological output to test for bilateralism. What this means is that if there is equal (bilateral) muscular function, for example, the flexor muscles of both forearms are functioning neurologically the same, then we can say that we have neutralized and balanced the body.

Up until now we have been talking about segmental alignment of the joints from a three-dimensional perspective. Now, let's put these concepts into the body as a living, breathing, moving human being. During movement, the body functionally divides itself into two units, passenger and locomotor. While there is motion and muscle action occurring in each function, the relative intensity is markedly different in the two units: Basically, the passenger unit is responsible only for its own postural integrity, and when structurally aligned on top of the locomotor unit, it has minimal demand. In fact, it should be a passive entity that is carried by the locomotor unit.

<u>Locomotor Unit</u>. The two lower limbs and pelvis are the anatomical segments that form the locomotor system. Fifty-seven muscles acting in a selective fashion control timeliness and magnitude of motion in each limb. The bony segments serve as levers. The pelvis has a dual role: 1) Mobile link between the two lower limbs, and 2) The bottom segment of the passenger unit that rides on the hips. As the locomotor unit carries the body to its desired location, each weight-bearing limb accomplishes four distinct functions:

1. A propulsive force is generated
2. Upright stability is maintained
3. The shock of floor impact at the onset of each stride is minimized
4. Energy is conserved by these functions being performed in a manner that reduces the amount of muscular effort required

This locomotor unit moves us forward along the surface of the earth, a process known as ambulation.

<u>The Passenger Unit</u>

The head, neck, trunk, and arms comprise the passenger

unit. Muscle action within the neck and trunk serve only to maintain neutral vertebral alignment. Arm swing is both active and passive, but the action does not appear essential to the normal gate pattern "(Perry, J. (1992). Gait analysis: Normal and pathological function. New York: McGraw-Hill). Together these four structures make up 70% of body weight. Here is where I disagree with common research. Most experts believe that within this composite mass lies the body's center of mass located just anterior to the tenth thoracic vertebra. As we discussed in chapter 10, the problem I see with this is that the center of mass SHOULD be located at the sacral level, if not as low as the superior border of the acetabulum because the COM is typically associated with the greatest amount of work being done in a structure; due to the fact that almost everyone who is analyzed structurally falls forward at the pelvic level in the Frontal Plane, the work would naturally displace itself higher above the pelvis in order to maintain stability in the body. This is why most people suffer from lower back pain because the passenger unit was not designed to take on the responsibility of holding up the entire body around gravity. As I explained, when we sit for long periods of time each day and throughout our lives, the lateral and medial stabilizers begin to shorten and become weak and therefore cannot hold the body aligned in the Frontal Plane. So, the natural tendency is for the workload to be transferred higher in the body and into the passenger unit in order to maintain some type of balance and homeostasis. However, conventional thought places the COM at a higher level, thereby presenting a long lever above the level of the hip joints. As a result, balance of the passenger unit would be even more dependent on the alignment of the lower limbs to move the base of support under the passenger unit's momentary center of gravity.

This passenger unit is not supposed to be active during ambulation. It is supposed to be passive and rest on top of the locomotor unit, which further supports my theory that the COM should be located more in the locomotor unit than in the passenger unit; one could say it is merely along for the ride. The passenger unit need only be engaged during activities that require finer motor acuity such as reaching and grasping.

What happens when the locomotor unit is either too weak to work or when it is prevented from doing its work? What we see is that as the strength and amount of work the locomotor unit can do diminishes, the role and responsibilities of the passenger unit increase in direct relation. If this role reversal exists and persists over an extended period of time, the size and/or strength of the passenger unit will increase to the extent that it will become bigger and heavier than its base, the locomotor unit, thus destabilizing the unit as a whole. The result is that gravity and ground reaction forces no longer meet in the center of the skeletal structure. This leaves both units vulnerable to external forces. The passenger unit now has no counteracting upward force to gravity's downward pulling force. What this means is that the passenger unit begins to topple over and move in the direction of gravity's pull, toward the ground. If left to continue, this situation will severely impact both the musculoskeletal and organ systems of the body. The result will be skeletal contortion, excessive strain and attrition on the bones, muscles and all soft tissue structures, generalized or chronic pain and discomfort, vulnerability to sudden and incapacitating pain or injury, as well as organ inefficiency and atrophy which includes cardiovascular disease, digestive disorders, migraine headaches, and chronic fatigue and sickness.

Walking forward on level ground is the basic locomotor pattern. A change in direction or gradient increases the demand placed upon the system to maintain this pattern. Running and various sports therefore present even greater needs (Perry, J. (1992). *Gait analysis: Normal and pathological function*).

Chapter 9

The Effects of Inactivity

Structural alignment provides for the maintenance of homeostasis: Active stability, shock absorption, energy conservation, and control and balance. Therefore, a lack of structural alignment provides for the misuse of the systems of our body. It dramatically affects our anatomy, physiology, psychology, and emotional well-being. The resultant symptoms are manifold and include: dysfunctional hypertrophy (due to chronic overuse), hypotrophy (due to under-use or neuropathy), fatigue, rigidity, a lack of mobility, instability, depression, migraine headaches, insomnia, inability to concentrate, cardiovascular disease(CVD), anxiety, pain, osteoporosis, arthritis, clumsiness, digestive disorders, decreased sex drive, and allergies, just to name a few.

Misalignment causes fatigue and inflexibility. Both make any type of movement difficult, and more than likely, painful. Pain will further decrease movement and eventually lead to inactivity. The fact that the human body is designed for movement is made more apparent when we examine the flip side of that statement: The human body was not designed for stillness or inactivity. So, when we stand still we are fighting our natural design, and putting our systems under great strain. The average workday for most people today is about 10 hours. And the majority of that time is usually spent sitting. Sitting is a very inactive state for the body to be in because it disengages the body's primary postural muscle group which is the iliopsoas. Nor are people necessarily active after work. So, for 10 plus hours each and every day, we fight our natural design and need for movement; we see the consequences of this every day in our clinic.

Specific changes that occur to the locomotor apparatus in response to inactivity and improper load bearing are: a decrease in oxygen supply due to decreased circulatory system efficiency, a loss of rapid motion and orthostatic tolerance, a decrease of postural sensory signals, and a lessened ability and finite motor acuity because of altered sensory input from both postural and dynamic musculature (Gluckman, *Muscle Balance and Function*).

The time frame for these responses to begin to take place is shown to be 24-72 hours (Joan Vernikos Ph.D., *Sitting Kills, Moving Heals*). The loss of postural cues, due to the deactivation of the antigravity muscles, also begin within this time frame. Since most of our clients have persisted in their postural misalignments for anywhere from 2 months to 40 years, the serious impact of such findings is quite breathtaking. The fact that postural technology can reverse these effects is even more astounding, demonstrating its power and tremendous ability to heal the human body.

The profound fact that the human body is designed for movement exposes the fundamental weakness of our passive western approach to medicine and healing. How can we attempt to help or heal an active entity passively? That would be like giving directions to an English speaker in French. For the body to understand and respond, the approach must be active. This is the power of postural technology. Postural technology asks the body to move in the manner the bones and the muscles tell us the body was designed to move. Hence, we are speaking its' language.

Let us take a good look at this language of movement and see where it comes from. Like all languages, it developed over time. So, let's begin with the evolution of the species Homo erectus – the erect man.

Man in motion: Millions of years ago man moved back over his hind limbs and stood erect for the first time. No longer would we move on all four limbs. From now on our two hind limbs would be our moving apparatus, and our two front limbs would be free to manipulate the environment and objects in the environments. This new way of being and moving was unique and it provided humans with numerous biomechanical advantages, but it would have large repercussions on our skeletal structure, specifically our spine and balance mechanisms; as well as our psychology, specifically our sense of vulnerability.

Our erect posture demanded that we balance on two feet. This meant that our spine had to shift from one single "C"-shaped curve supported on either end, to a more cushioning and absorbing "S"- shaped curve supported on only one end. Standing erect on two feet also shifted our center of gravity further away from the ground thereby changing the relationship our parts have to each other, as well as their relationships the body as a whole and with the external environment. How all this made us feel as a species is debatable, yet it is our contention, based on Darwin's Theory of Evolution, that, psychologically, we are a species based in fear. We fear that we will be destroyed because we know how easily it can happen, given the atavistic awareness of how it was when we were on all fours with our internal organs were protected by being closer to the earth's surface and more hidden from possible predators.

The combination of our erect posture and design to move with today's modern, highly technological society has proven disastrous to our health and well-being. We are forced to misuse our skeletal and muscular systems by sitting, wearing clothes and shoes, which basically disengaging ourselves proprioceptively from our environment, in order to preserve our ability to survive and provide shelter, food and protection to ourselves and our family.

Charles Darwin explains the effect of habit and the use and disuse of parts as it relates to the evolution of our medical system: We have a built-in inclination for the preservation of favorable individual differences and variations, and for the destruction of those which are injurious and threaten our survival. It would then follow that it would also be instinctual for humans to seek out methods to assist in preservation of these favorable differences and in basic protection. Back in the Ice Age this instinct led to creating fire, and tools such as the spear, to defend against predators. Nowadays, the threats have changed faces. In place of the saber-toothed tiger, and freezing cold, our challenge is inactivity and its intimate link with technology. Our solutions have also changed. They have gone from being primarily active to passive, and because they are passive, they lead to the preservation, rather than the eradication, of the injurious adaptations that our cultural patterns of inactivity or incorrect activity have led us too (Darwin).

In a nutshell, we mostly sit, and our ancestors did not. Sitting deactivates our antigravity muscles. This state of inactivity alters the coordination of responses emitted and received from the central nervous system, which controls all bodily function. This is why Postural Alignment Technology™ is so necessary today. The following are 4 basic side postures; which one are you?

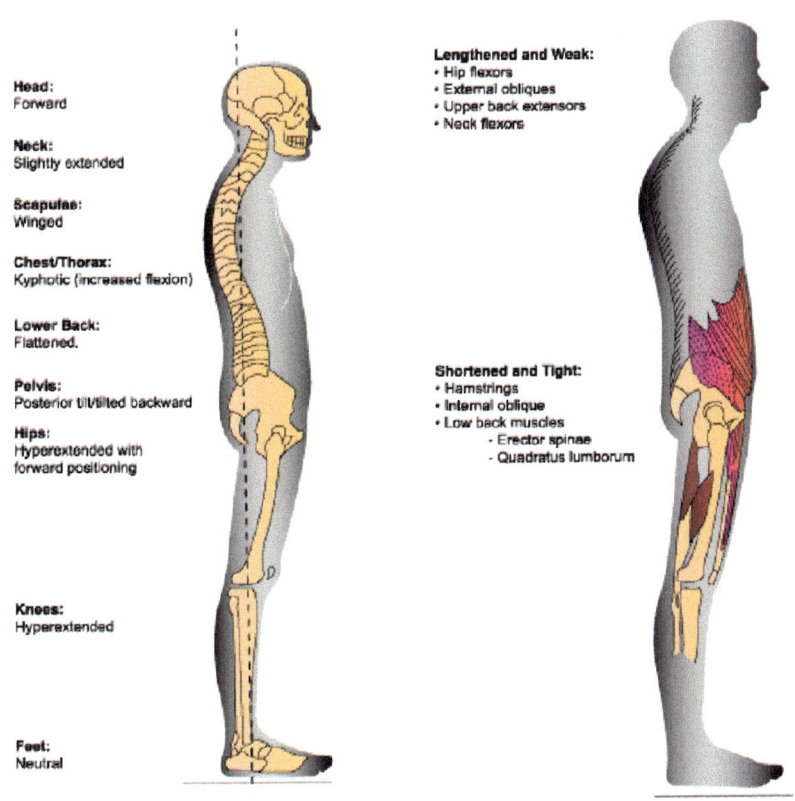

Kyphosis is associated with an increase curve of the thoracic spine. Along with this, a slightly posterior pelvic tilt is seen along with a reduced lumbar curve and a forward head position. The client will show a hunched over posture with a depressed chest.

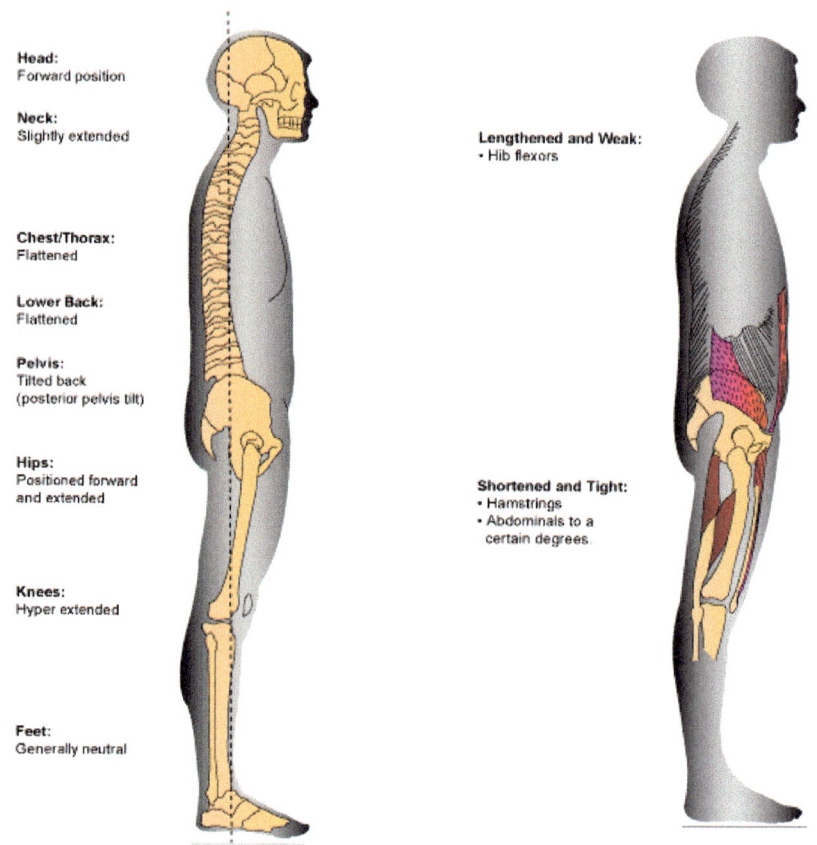

A flat back is when very little or no lumbar curve is present. There will pretty much always be a posterior pelvic tilt in a neutral position. Occasionally due to the position of the hip it can be difficult to fully straighten the knees when standing.

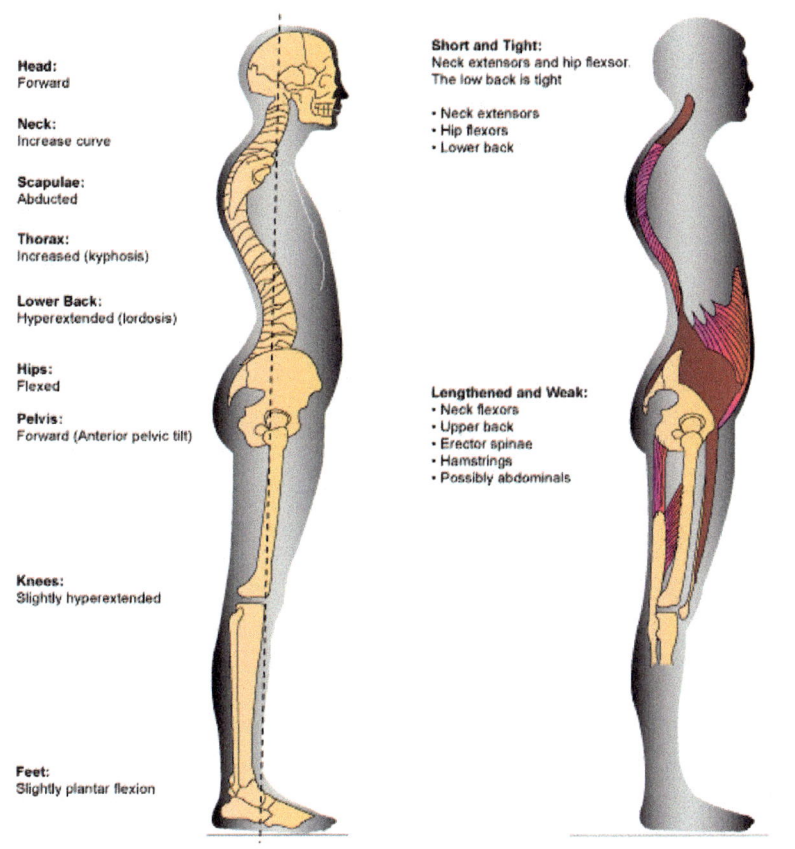

A sway-back posture can be seen with a neutral or posterior pelvic tilt with the hip almost rolled upward to the front. The client shows a relaxed posture, leaning backwards with the upper body.

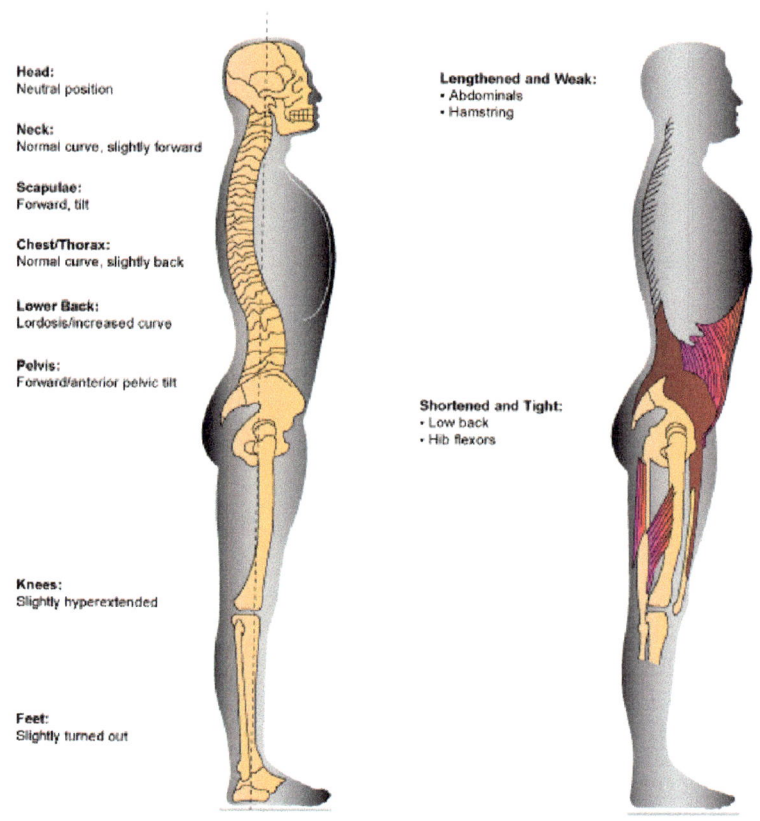

The Military type posture is more like what correct posture should look like. It is characterized by an increased curve in the lumbar spine of lower back and an anterior pelvic tilt. The client shows a posture in which the chest is pushed forward, shoulders retracted, or pulled back, and load-bearing joints aligned vertically.

Chapter 10

Postural Alignment Technology™

I created Symmetry to fill a void in a system that is more worried about codes and prescriptions than care and results. Symmetry was created to help fill the unanswered questions that so many people have when it comes to their pain. We all have our answers, but we fail to give solutions. When medicine first began the doctors used to make house calls. They had a rapport with their patients. They got to know them intimately and spent the time necessary to make sure their care was beyond adequate. Today, we have to work on volume or

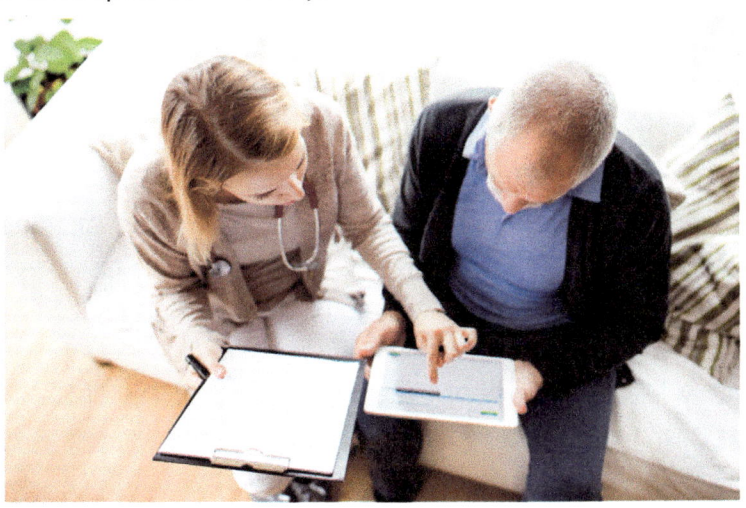

we don't get paid enough to run a business. As practitioners, we know the limitations of our system and we do the best to work within that system, however, I think we can all agree that the system isn't as effective as it should be. Why? Because there really isn't an incentive for people to actually get better. Treatments consist primarily of "in-clinic" care, and our effort isn't on what the patient should be doing at home to enhance or continue the healing process. Providers don't get paid for that. As service providers, the issue we have always had is that if we are not in the office, then we are not getting paid, and therefore we become slaves to our job, and eventually it tears us down, and our service suffers.

Recently a new client came into our clinic and began telling me his story that I have heard more than a thousand times in my career. He had a herniated disc for which the doctors recommended surgery and he obliged. Several years later, the same area was affected and to make things worse, he developed herniations in his neck as well. The doctor told him that one had nothing to do with the other. He refused to have another surgery and decided to try other avenues, all of which failed. But the one common theme that he expressed, like so many others, was that he wanted to know what he could do himself on a daily basis that would possibly assist him in become healthy. People are starting to change their paradigms about healing, and more than ever are willing to participate in their care. The internet has helped change this as people are realizing that the success of pain relief isn't what we once thought. The stats are there for everyone to see. I once read an article where a doctor was asked what his definition of a successful surgery was. His answer was that success was based upon the patient feeling no worse after the surgery.

Symmetry's number one philosophy is based upon a "client's participation" and the support they need to be accountable – all of this continues OUTSIDE of our office. Our philosophy lies solely on the education of a person to make long-term changes in their everyday habits and have them check in with us every other week. This does two things to ensure success:

1. When our clients get better, they understand that THEY did the work and view their return to health more as a personal achievement.

2. As a business, we no longer have to position our pricing on a "per visit" basis, but rather as a "holistic" program that involves both in-office treatment and at-home support. It is our belief that the focus of health care should be 90% education and support and 10% in-office treatment. It is also our belief that with proper instruction, our body has an amazing capacity to heal itself.

So how does the Postural Alignment Technology™ work? As I mentioned previously, the idea behind Symmetry is to give practitioners the tools to be able to better engage with their clients and help them realize that what they do is making a difference beyond just making them feel better. We have proven that people more than ever want a tangible explanation of why they are feeling better. We have all pledged as practitioners that our number one goal is to help our clients to become healthy and pain-free, which ironically would make them less reliant on us, which at first blush looks like decreased revenue. However, what if you could get people better, more quickly while helping them to feel empowered? I guarantee that you will reap the benefits.

Postural Alignment Technology™ really boils down to simplicity.

KISS. What I learned from Geoff Gluckman that revolutionized my way of thinking about the body was when he talked about the planes of motion. But it was when he described how to assess the body around the planes of motion that really triggered my enthusiasm. When I worked at the Egoscue Method, what we really did was try and assess which muscles were over-engaged and pick exercises that addressed those specific areas. This really is no different than any other therapy. However, because we didn't work with planes, it was impossible to assess which tight muscles to work on first. What Geoff explained was that when you are subjectively looking at a body, instead of looking to see what part is out of alignment, look to see from which plane the part of the body is misaligned. So, if you see an elevated hip for example, the observation is obviously that the hips are not level, but the correct assessment would be that the hip is elevated away from the transverse plane. Why? Because in order for the pelvis to rotate correctly in the transverse plane, the hips must be level, much like the relationship between a tire and an axel. If there isn't a right angel relationship, then the tire won't rotate correctly. When you look at the body what you are first recognizing is the imbalances that stand out the most. Understanding what plane they are deviating away from, is crucial to understanding which exercise to choose to correct the specific deviation, which I will talk about later in this chapter. However,

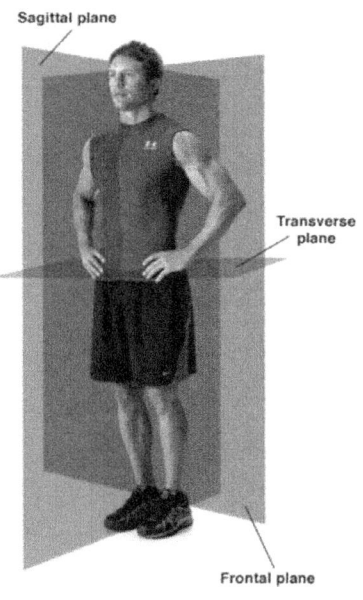

what needs to be understood here is that wherever there is an imbalance, the movement within the plane it is deviating away from will then be compromised.

As I mentioned previously, most practitioners do not take pictures of their clients. This is one of the most important tools for explaining the AlignSmart™ system. Because the entire body is taken under consideration, it is extremely valuable to use one's pictures to map out their disparities and compensations in showing them the cause behind their pain. It is a very rare circumstance where a traditional practitioner will take a full body shot and is usually only associated with research. In most cases, an x-ray or MRI will be taken to isolate the "painful" area and used primarily for explanation. The main purpose for our use of pictures is to make the client aware of the imbalances that he/she has developed over the years and to initiate the steps towards an everyday assessment when looking in the mirror each morning. The problem with most people is the fact that there has been no education about the fundamental principles of the human body as it relates to posture, gravity and pain. Therefore, there is no awareness or insight to the predictors of pain because we do not know what to look for and more importantly what to expect. Our job is to explain the physics of one's body in much the same way a structural engineer would explain the physics behind a building or the design of a car. They must be given a tangible comparison in order to create a clear understanding to the physics behind any structure as it relates to gravity. Pictures are the greatest tools in showing the comparison to "what should be" and "what is" in terms of a structural blueprint and how it relates to their current condition. It is the first step to the understanding of the cause of their pain. It is commonly referred as a "subjective evaluation".

The subjective visual assessment analysis of the human body must begin from a broad perspective. So often the obvious is overlooked because we have tunnel vision in dealing with pain. Therefore, most analyses often lead to a misdiagnosis and often mistreatment. You must view one's body like the puzzles that have no shape until you adapt your vision to the right dimension and suddenly you see a shape form right in

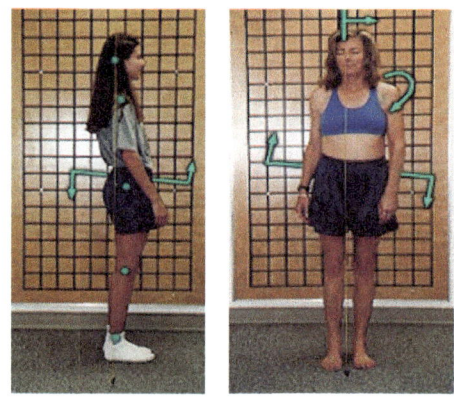

front of you. Therefore, the order of the visual evaluation should be to first find the greatest disparity then continue until you see the least. Remember, you are looking for anything that is skewed from right angles around three-dimensional space first. It is what we refer to as "red flags". Have someone take a few pictures of your posture; front, side and back. Take a look at the following list and see if you have any of these visual imbalances:

    1. Feet everted, inverted (pronated or supinated).

    2. Hand forward or rounded more than the other.

3. Forward rotation of the pelvis.

4. Upper torso rotation (one arm in front more than the other).

5. Scapulae protracted, retracted, or elevated.

6. One hip higher than the other.

7. More space between one arm and the torso versus the other.

8. Knees internal or external or one knee internal and the other external.

9. Knees varus or valgus (bow-legged or knock-kneed).

10. Offset of the torso.

11. Offset of the head.

12. Knee flexion or hyperextension.

13. Forward displacement of the pelvis or head from the side view.

14. Take notice of muscular asymmetries such as one calf larger than the other, etc.

Now, let's take a look at the same list above and ask yourself which plane these deviations occur away from. The list below defines this:

1. Feet everted, inverted (pronated or supinated): **Sagittal**

2. Hand forward or rounded more than the other: **Frontal**

3. Forward rotation of the pelvis: **Frontal**

4. Upper torso rotation (one arm in front more than the other): **Frontal**

5. Scapulae protracted, retracted: **Frontal**

6. Scapulae elevated: **Transverse**

7. One hip higher than the other: **Transverse**

8. More space between one arm and the torso versus the other: **Sagittal**

9. Knees medial or external or one knee medial and the other external: **Sagittal**

10. Knees varus or valgus: **Sagittal**

11. Offset of the torso: **Sagittal**

12. Offset of the head: **Sagittal**

13. Knee flexion or hyperextension: **Frontal**

14. Forward displacement of the pelvis or head: **Frontal**

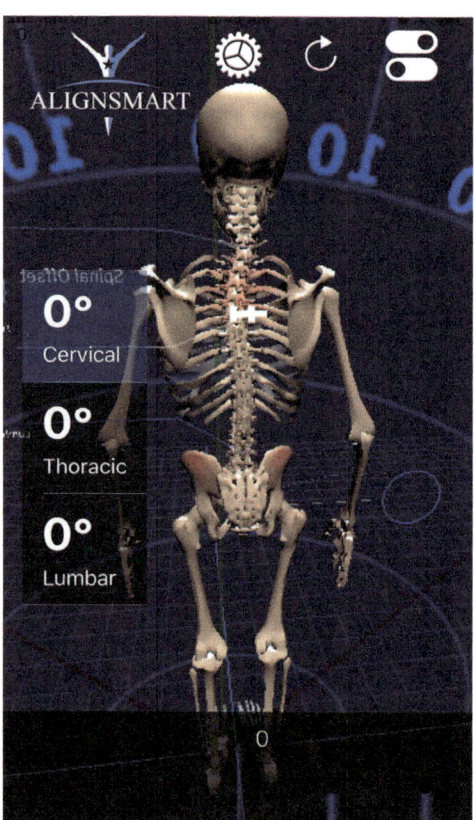

A spinal offset is an example of a sagittal deviation

As a practitioner, this is the point where we can really impress our clients. With each evaluation, you will begin to realize certain patterns that are fairly typical of most individuals. These are what we call "rules of thumb". Rules of thumb are derived from the "red flag" analysis and are formally known as the righting reflexes. This will be discussed further in the "objective evaluation" section, but should be noted here as well. These rules of thumb correspond with the "righting reflexes" stated earlier in the book. For example, if one of the obvious disparities you see in your client is a left shoulder elevated, then it can be assumed that the right hip will be elevated. Why? Because most compensations occur from the pelvic level due to the inability to stabilize around the foundation of one's body. If the right hip is elevated, there will be a typical response for the spine to laterally shift away from the elevation. Because the position of the head must be directly in line with the COM in the sagittal plane, a "righting response" will occur within the left side of the body, thus triggering the trapeziums and corresponding muscles to pull the head back into alignment. This is what I call the "Cross-Compensation Effect™". This applies to all other planar compensations as well. Here is a list of typical patterns among "normal" people when seen for the first time as well as some general rules:

- Typically, an elevated Iliac Crest (IC) will compensate for the posterior angle of the PSIS-ASIS on the opposite side. However, with athletes it is typically the opposite. The elevated IC is usually the posterior one.

- Shoulder disparities almost always come from pelvic disparities.

- If the Iliac Crest on one hip is elevated, the opposite side scapulae will usually elevate to compensate.

- If the Iliac Crest and the Scapulae on the same side are both elevated, then the lumbar spine is shifting towards the elevated Ilium.

- The body will typically compensate in a way that repositions the head in relationship to the center-point of the pelvis, thus maintaining equilibrium within the body. I.e.:

- If the Greater Trochanter (GT) is displaced forward 4", the upper torso must stay back, and the head will reposition directly vertical to the GT.
- If a hip is elevated it will laterally shift the spine and the head will pull back into alignment centered over the pelvis.
- If the pelvis is rotated left to right, then the upper torso will counter-rotate right to left and the head will rotate back left to right to keep the head balanced within the sagittal plane.
- External knees in a sedentary man usually indicate a posterior PSIS-ASIS on the same side.
- External knees on an athlete usually indicate an anterior tilt of the pelvic associated with tight hip flexors.
- Medial knees in women usually indicate a posterior PSIS-ASIS angle on the same side and very weak hip flexors.
- Excess body weight does affect the integrity of a structure, but does not restrict one from ridding themselves from pain.
- Medial knees are indicative of weakness in the frontal and sagittal planes.
- One knee external and one knee neutral or medial indicates a transverse disparity.
- Runners primarily deviate from the frontal plane.
- Most athletes are typically more misaligned in the transverse plane. This is due to the fact that most sports are one-side dominant.
- Large inverted/abducted feet and a widened stance

are a result of an inability to hold the pelvis in the frontal plane. This reaction occurs as a compensation to widen the support base to decrease the responsibility in the pelvic region.

- Pigeon-toed athletes are faster than duck-footed athletes. This is due to the fact that our visual assessment of feet that appear pigeon-toed are really aligned. It is not the norm, but from a physics perspective, the more all toes are pointing straight ahead, the greater push-off you can get when running straight ahead. It's called force vectors.
- Thoracic inflexibility corresponds with inflexible hamstrings.
- Everted (pronated) feet indicate a posterior tilt of the same side.
- 95% of all normal active children under the age of 9 have an anterior tilt of 10 degrees.
- Women tend to hyperextend at the knees more than men.
- There is a genetic component to some structural abnormalities.
- Valgus knees are more a result of structural compensations, whereas varus knees tend to be more genetic in nature.
- Form precedes function, in our society.
- Nearly 100% of the population has scoliosis. HOWEVER, the majority have the functional type.

Okay, back to the process. I came up with the AlignSmart™ system through a series of trial and error. When I first started Symmetry back in 1997 I was still performing the basic Egoscue method. Not really knowing what I was doing, but still having fairly good success. When I went through the Gluckman series, it painted a much clearer picture for me in understanding the dimensional relationships of the body around gravity. But, when I started measuring, it changed the game. By measuring every joint in the body and being able to compare quantitatively how it is positioned against the true form, revealed relationships that could not only be explained, but monitored. In 2003 when I found the programmer for my first software system, I was forced to figure out all of the relationships with the measurements and factors I was using during my sessions. Up to that point, I had a pretty good understanding of what I was doing, but it still wasn't as precise as I wanted it to be. I would measure, take a look at the overall values, and then start writing down exercises that I knew would correct each disparity and then try and sequence them appropriately. The problem with this is that I would still tend to pick the same general pool of exercises because the brain (mine in any case) can only hold so much pertinent information at one time. So, the routines ended up looking more or less the same all the time. However, I was still able to monitor the changes in measurements with my clients from session to session, which I found to be a huge advantage regardless of whether my routines were perfect or not.

When we started to create the first software, my wife suggested I write down every factor I used with each client. The following chart is part of what I came up with after three months of breaking down, apart, and putting it all together. The bottom line of this method is to be as focused as possible, with a sequence of corrective exercises that best fit not only the structural deviations of each client, but the emotional/cognitive factors to make sure that they will be consistent in doing the routines in between each appointment.

This chart is the conclusion of years of dealing with the human

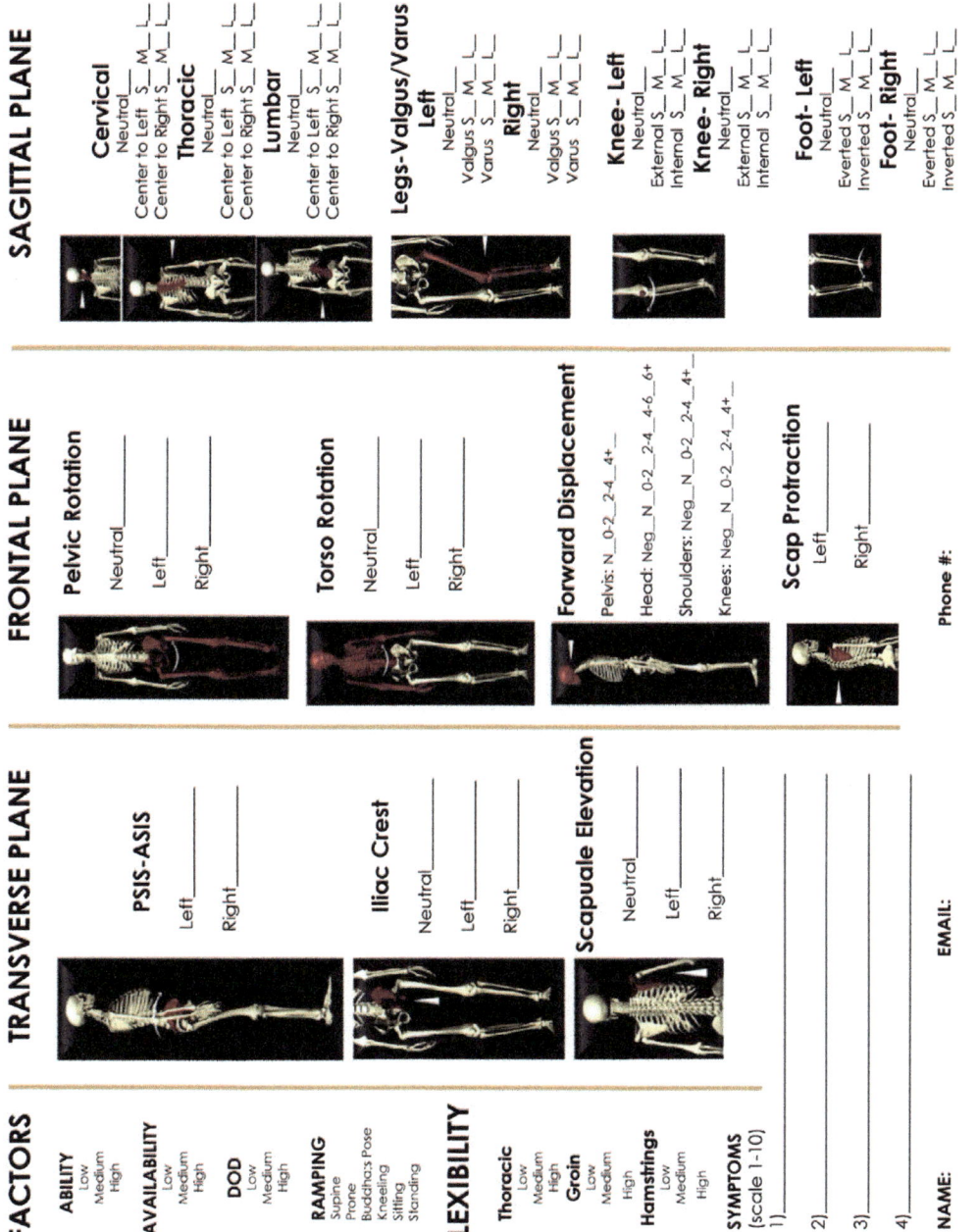

being. If you look at the chart closely, these are all the factors that are associated with choosing the most effective exercises to correct the current pattern evaluated and in the best sequence possible. And this is why I have a patent on this system. I don't care what healthcare profession you are talking about, there is a sequence to what they do regarding their treatment, at least there should be. However, the biggest issue is that since each evaluation is not quantified, then the practitioner CANNOT teach the sequence to anyone else due to relying on instinct only. Ultimately, the treatment becomes almost exclusively about diminishing pain or symptoms, and at the end of the day the treatment becomes a series of educated guesses. So, if a client isn't relieved of pain after a few sessions, then that client won't come back, because the practitioner has not given them enough evidence to convince them to stay in treatment.

When I have a new client if front of me, I literally tell them that if their main objective in coming to our office is to rid themselves of pain, then they are in the wrong clinic. Our main objective is putting their bodies back into proper form, thus proper function, and the result will be a decrease or ridding or their issues. Simple. Because I have a method to explain how the body is changing and how we must unravel years of compensation first, before we can strengthen them completely, I have the ability to coach my clients through the entire process. I have had clients stick with us for the full three-month program and on the last session finally get out of pain due to the complexity of their compensation patterns. But they stick with us, because I can show them where their bodies were, where they are now, and where I know they will go. It's physics, and as long as I have a proactive client, I know I have someone that will beat their years of chronic pain. It just takes time, education, commitment and motivation. Most therapies don't work simply because people don't spend enough time in the process to allow the body to heal! So, if you were to have evidence that you were going in the right direction, I certainly know that you would be more willing to stay engaged in the process. Yes, some of our clients are so badly compensated that they need more than three months to heal, but we stay with them until they do. This should be the healthcare model we all engage in.

Okay, so let's take a closer look at the previous chart. Every item on this page is used to generate a specific sequence of corrective exercises (I will talk more about our "exercises" in a bit, because the word "exercise" is deceiving). Each factor and each measurement combine to create the ultimate sequence to combat the current layer of compensation evaluated. Here they are defined:

1. **Ability:** The ability of a client refers to the "kinesthetic awareness" a person displays as it pertains to being able to follow directions with the exercises suggested. If a client has "Low Ability", this means that they do not have the awareness to perform complex exercises correctly and will more than likely perform it incorrectly at home. What are you?

2. **Availability:** The routines can be sequenced either in 10, 20 or 30-minute segments. This is determined by your willingness to consistently commit to performing the routine daily. We have proven over a 21-year career that people will NOT consistently participate in ANY program if it is more than 30 minutes at a time per day. What would you be

willing to commit to?

3. Degree of Difficulty (DOD): This refers to how hard you want to work in a routine. A "Low" DOD means that the majority of exercises will be passive, whereas the "High" level will be exercises that require a high-level of effort or work. A lot of this however is determined by the symptoms of a client as well. How hard can you be pushed?

4. Ramping: This factor refers to the position that a client finishes their routine. For example, if you choose "Supine", then ALL the exercises will be on the floor, on the back. As I previously mentioned in chapter 6, it literally takes on average 1 year to get from the floor to standing from the time we are born. This is the ramping process that the brain has to develop around in order to connect the neuromuscular dots. When a client comes in for each appointment, we must determine if they indeed can get to a standing position without the overall compensation correction being negatively affected. I know this sounds a bit funny, because anyone can stand; however, if we add more and more levers around gravity, and the body cannot handle the load due to the amount of compensation, then the body will default back to its "known" or "remembered" holding patterns, which will render the sequence null and void. This is one my biggest criticisms of most "physical" therapies or training sessions. Most people cannot hold their own body weight correctly around gravity, so when you try and treat or train the body in a dysfunctional position, standing being the most prevalent, all you are doing is strengthening this dysfunction. Thus, no new patterns are engrained.

5. Flexibility: There are three main areas for flexibility:

Thoracic, Groin, and Hamstring. This is an overall assessment of a client's flexibility which will ultimately determine which exercise they can perform or not. Check out the steps below and assess your own flexibility:

a. Thoracic:

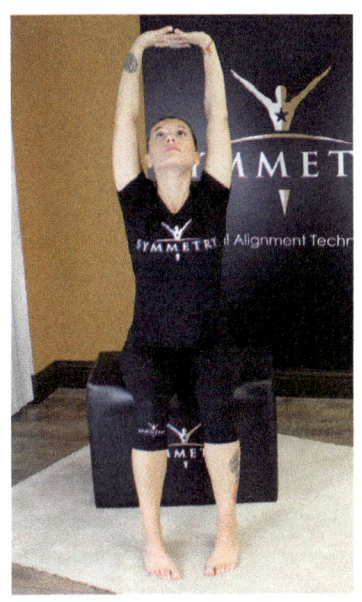

i. Sit on a chair with your knees bent at 90 degrees.

ii. Interlace your hands pushing your palms away. While locking your elbows, raise your arms overhead and behind your head as far as possible without leaning your torso backwards.

iii. Assess your flexibility in three categories: Low, Medium, or High.

- Low: You have an extremely difficult time locking your arms and pulling them to the front of your face.

- Medium: You have a reasonable ability to pull your arms back and can get your arms parallel to your head.

- High: You have no problem pulling your arms behind your head.

b. Groin:

i. Sit on a chair with your knees bent at 90 degrees.

ii. Place an ankle to the opposite knee (Both sides). The leg that has the lowest flexibility is the one you

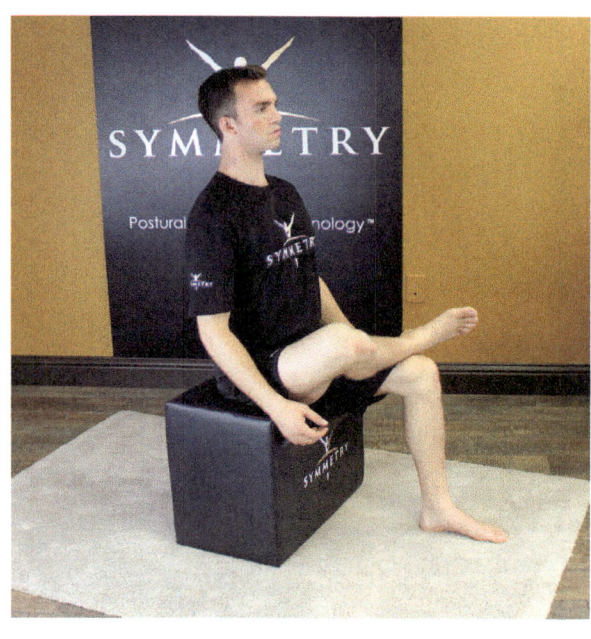

record.

- Low: You have an extremely difficult time pushing your knee away and have a hard time even getting the ankle to the knee.

- Medium: You have a reasonable ability to push your knee away.

- High: You have no problem pushing your knee away.

c. Hamstrings

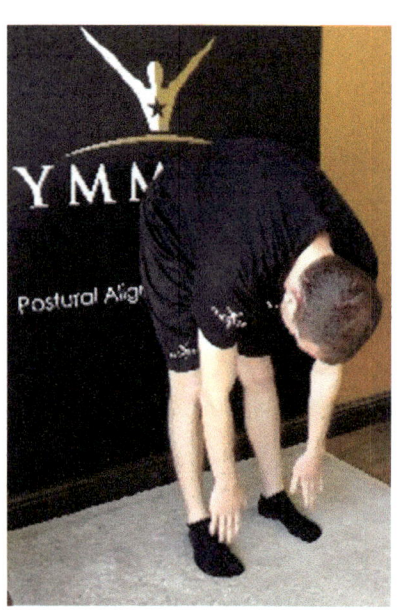

i. Stand with your feet hip width

ii. While keeping your legs locked, slowly bend at the waist and try and touch your toes.

- Low: Client has an extremely difficult time bending down and can barely reach their knees.

- Medium: Client has a reasonable ability to reach past their knees and to their ankles.

- High: Client has no problem touching their toes or the floor.

6. Symptoms: Remember, we really are not dealing with symptoms; we are dealing with the cause of the symptoms. However, if someone has been injured by a contact accident and they are in acute pain, this program is probably inappropriate at this juncture and may not be suitable until one has stabilized the injured area. Remember, we are focusing on getting rid of the pain by understanding how to treat the cause. Just by evaluating your client correctly, you will more than likely be able to accurately guess where your client's discomfort is located. However, we still need to understand where and what the symptoms are so that we do not exacerbate them and can at least monitor the pain throughout the course of treatment.

It is very important that you do your best to correctly label the pain intensity using the Mankoski Pain Scale, for each exercise is connected with a specific category for the symptom so as to avoid any exercises that might be contraindicated with the pain. The symptom level will mainly be important when the pain levels are 5 and higher, and the position or activity of the exercise will negatively affect the pain level. For example, if one has severe back pain of 7 from a herniated disc, and their hips are elevated and the angles skewed, then you will not want to rotate the spine even though the evaluation calls for it. In this instance, you would find exercises that could indirectly address these compensations or choose other indirect methods of addressing this disparity.

Therefore, the client's symptoms will be one of the last factors to potentially alter the ramping and degree of difficulty of a routine. It has the ability to override the length and intensity of a routine. In other words, if you have a highly motivated, highly available, high ability client who has intense pain, then you will more than likely keep the ramping at an even keel and keep them on the floor. However, you also must understand that the Mankoski Pain Scale is also used to categorize areas that might not be symptomatic, but might have a limitation. Factors associated with this category are past injuries, surgeries, permanent fixtures such as rods, fusions, joint replacements, etc., and current diagnoses.

Here is the scale. Assess your own pain and give it a number:

Mankoski Pain Scale
Copyright © 1995, 1996, 1997 Andrea Mankoski. All rights reserved.
Right to copy with attribution freely granted.

1. Pain Free. No Medication Needed.

2. Very Minor Annoyance. Occasional Minor Twinges, No Medication Needed.

3. Minor annoyance. Occasional strong twinges. No medication needed.

4. Annoying enough to be distracting. Mild painkillers are effective. (Aspirin, Ibuprofen.)

5. Can be ignored if you are really involved in your work, but still distracting. Mild painkillers relieve pain for 3-4 hours.

6. Can't be ignored for more than 30 minutes. Mild painkillers reduce pain for 3-4 hours.

7. Can't be ignored for any length of time, but you can still go to work and participate in social activities. Stronger painkillers (Codeine, Vicodin) reduce pain for 3-4 hours.

8. Makes it difficult to concentrate, interferes with sleep. You can still function with effort. Stronger painkillers are only partially effective. Strongest painkillers relieve pain (OxyContin, Morphine)

9. Physical activity severely limited. You can read and converse with effort. Nausea and dizziness set in as factors of pain. Stronger painkillers are minimally effective. Strongest painkillers reduce pain for

3-4 hours.

10. Unable to speak. Crying out or moaning uncontrollably - near delirium. Strongest painkillers are only partially effective.

11. Unconscious. Pain makes you pass out. Strongest painkillers are only partially effective.

7. Measurements: This is the crux of our AlignSmart™ Technology system. Without the measurements, we have no system. Without measurements, no one has a true system. Without a system, no one can evidence or replicate the sequence needed to correct a problem. Without a sequence, then what a practitioner ultimate does is focus on ridding you of your pain, which as we have discussed, is the end by-product of your years of compensation.

So, here is how it works. The body as we have explained works in three plane. You have to hold yourself balanced in each plane using intrinsic muscles, so that you can

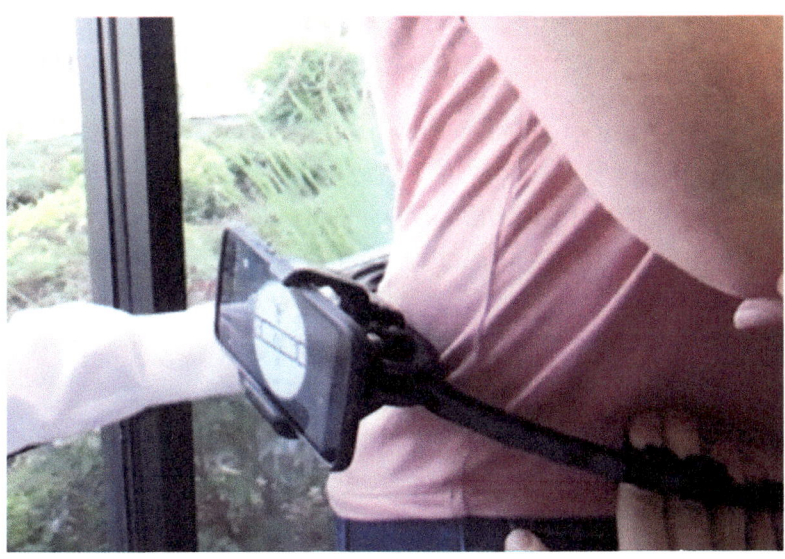

effectively move within each plane using dynamic muscles. The skeleton therefore, is strategically designed to support specific muscles that are attached in such a way to optimize this function. We are the only clinic that I know of that does not use muscle testing as our main source of evaluation. What we do is measure 21 bony landmarks which determine, or better yet, map out the static neuromuscular holding

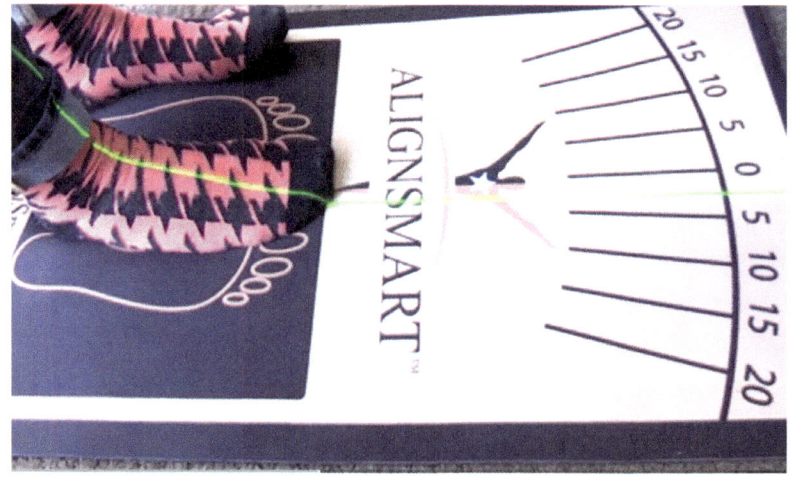

pattern around the force of gravity. We do this using our patented Postural Alignment Tool™ and the AlignSmart™ Technology system to quantify these measurements. Remember that ultimately, pain is derived from the **inability** for muscles to hold and move bones correctly. If we can understand these patterns, then we can generate relational information from the planes that tell us how to correct these patterns.

So, now you are probably asking, "How do I measure myself?" The answer is, "You can't!", effectively anyway. This is the problem with "self-help" books. They can only help you to a certain degree, and then they become ineffective. If you want to be measured, give us a call and we'll locate a Symmetry AlignSmart™ Professional near you!

Chapter 11

The Exercises

This is where the rubber meets the road. In today's physical health world there are so many philosophies behind getting people strong and out of pain. I hear almost daily where a new client will come in and tell me that their doctor or healthcare provider has suggested highly that they increase their "core" workout to help strengthen their back. In typical rehab therapy, most of the exercises prescribed are focused on the pain area itself. Another is "I was told to get back in the gym and start strength training". At Symmetry, we don't encourage these practices initially. As we explained previously, if your frame is bent, it doesn't matter what car you drive or what you "fix" if you are still out of alignment. I had mentioned in chapter 1 that going into my senior year at SDSU I went from a 200-pound bench press to 300 pounds. What I didn't explain to you was that every time I went into the weight room, my left hip angle was posterior, my right ilium was elevated, my pelvis was rotated left to right, and my right shoulder was very protracted and elevated. These were just some of my issues, but what I wasn't told was that I had to prepare my structural body before any of my activities. I was told to build my core strength and to stretch as much as I could. We'll, I'm here to tell you that I did both to the extreme. But it wasn't too soon into my senior year that I quickly realized that every time I stretched before a game, I would get injured. In 2006, I had the opportunity to follow Az Hakim when he re-signed with the Detroit Lions. He introduced me to their strength and conditioning coach Bert Hill. I remember Bert asking me once what I thought about his linemen stretching before a game or practice. I told him I didn't like it the way it is approached typically. He agreed stating many references to research that indicated that stretching before activity actually caused more injuries. So, he told me that they did more "warm-up" drills than traditional stretching. I didn't go into my theories with him at the time, but if I had I would have given the opinion that he was wrong in doing so. You see, I am not against stretching per say, I am against stretching in and of itself, by itself. What I mean by this is that I found out half-way through my senior season that when I did concentrate on stretching prior to a game, I usually had some type of injury that game. So, I too, began just performing some general warm-up drills, such as wind-sprints, to loosen up my body. But stretching is not the problem. Knowing what I know now, I realize that what people do when they just concentrate on stretching, is to lengthen a tight muscle. But when you understand physics and compensation patterns, what you will end up realizing yourself, is that when you stretch out your tight muscles, you are in fact stretching out the muscles that your brain has recruited to help stabilize an imbalanced body. So many times, I get a client that will come in and tell me that they had a bad reaction to a massage. Same thing. If you understand the main component of any typical passive treatment model such as massage, acupuncture or chiropractic, you are dealing with a passive client lying on a table and getting rubbed, needled or adjusted. The common denominator is a "release" occurs, which will feel very good initially. But quite soon after, your muscular default pattern will reengage due to the fact that you did nothing to strengthen the change that just occurred. So, when you release tight muscles and don't strengthen the imbalance that caused the tightness in the first place, your brain says "no" and pulls you back into protection mode.

So, do you think the type of exercises matter when trying to figure out how to rid someone of pain? You bet. When people ask what type of exercises we use at Symmetry, we usually explain that our system is most like scientific yoga, in a sense. Yoga primarily uses isometric exercises, which are the best form of exercises to change posture, but there is no measuring, and therefore, everyone goes through the same sequence. We get a lot of clients who come in injured from doing yoga. However, if we taught yoga instructors the AlignSmart™ system, it would be a game changer. Soon enough.

In the meantime, let's dive deeper into the different types of exercises and see what each one should be primarily used for.

> **1) Passive**- a passive exercise is one that has **no work** associated with it. It is typically a releasing exercise or a resting exercise such as the Static Floor or Wall Groin Stretch. This would be considered a static stretching exercise where the body is positioned on the floor using multiple reference points to allow the weight of the body to act upon a joint or joints. Staying in this passive position long enough allows for the brain to disengage due to no work being done, and also for compensated muscle groups to "let go", allowing for temporary relief.
>
> **2) Isometric**- an isometric exercise is one that provides **work without movement** and describes the majority of Symmetry

Postures. These exercises can include more isometric stretching such as the Piriformis Crossovers, or strengthening such as the regular Piriformis Stretch. Isometric exercises are considered the most appropriate for changing postural misalignment because they most directly influence the intrinsic musculature due to the fact that intrinsic muscles do not change length with external force. Therefore, to move the body dynamically will NOT change the postural position of the body but only enhance the compensation patterns already developed. Here are the benefits of isometric training (breakingmuscle.com):

I. **One of the main benefits of isometric training is that the body is able to activate nearly all the available motor units - something that is usually very difficult to do.** Back in the 1950s, researchers Hettinger and Muller found a single daily effort of two-thirds of a person's maximum effort exerted for six seconds at a time for ten weeks increased strength about 5% per week, while Clark and associates demonstrated static strength continued to increase even after the conclusion of a five-week program of isometric exercises.

II. Another benefit of isometric training is simply the amount of time spent performing an exercise. Consider an exercise like the bench press. It may take one to two seconds to perform with each joint angle only being trained for short periods of time. In contrast, an exercise that mimics the bench press, like a press against pins at the sticking point of the lift, may be performed for several seconds. **In other words, if you**

have a problem at a particular joint angle in a lift, you can do targeted isometrics to quickly overcome your problems.

III. Given that you can perform isometrics with little equipment and a relatively short timeframe, you'd think they'd be far more popular in the training world. So why aren't they mainstream? For starters, there's no denying the commercial aspect. With isometrics, there's no valuable equipment to sell. Secondly, there has been some selective use of the science involved in isometric research.

IV. **Like all good training methods, you need to know how and when to apply isometrics, and how to overcome whatever shortfalls it has.** Every system has holes in it, but our job is to explain to you how to overcome it. Potential decreases in muscle elasticity and speed of movement are easy to overcome with the use of relaxation and stretching methods such we use in Symmetry.

V. Research has shown that because of the reduced blood flow during prolonged muscle tension, numerous growth factors remain in the muscle tissue longer and actually stimulate muscle growth. Doing a higher number of contractions increases strength, while holding contractions longer increases muscle mass. (https://draxe.com/isometric-exercises/)

VI. Convenient style of training at any place and at almost any time. Isometric exercises can provide a source of strength training at any place and whenever you feel like it. While there is some equipment that you may find useful for isometric exercises at the gym, you can perform these exercises without any equipment at all, making it very convenient while helping you maintain your fitness goals.

VII. May be helpful to someone who is healing from an injury. Isometric exercises provide a source of strength training without the impact that more complex exercises may require. For example, if you have a shoulder injury, a physical therapist may recommend some isometric exercises that stabilize the shoulder and maintain strength in that area so that the recovery is faster.

VIII. May help lower blood pressure. The Mayo Clinic notes that a recent study has shown that isometric exercises may also help naturally lower your blood pressure since exercising at higher intensities can cause a dramatic increase in your blood pressure, specifically during the activity. Regardless, it is important to check with your doctor before beginning isometric exercises if you have high blood pressure or any heart problems. Also, please note that isometric exercise can also increase blood pressure during performance; however, a regular exercise program generally helps reduce blood pressure. A study conducted by the Division of Cardiology at University Health Network in Toronto, Canada suggests that isometric exercise training in young and old participants may produce reductions in blood pressure. In this case, isometric exercise training protocols typically consisted of four sets of two-minute handgrip or leg contractions sustained at 20–50 percent of maximal voluntary contraction, with each set separated by a rest period of 1–4 min. Training was usually completed three to five times per week for 4–10 weeks. Improvements in the regulation of heart rate and blood pressure have been reported. Some key things to remember: never hold your breath or strain during any training exercise, as this may cause a dangerous rise in blood pressure.

IX. Relieve depression. American physician and cardiologist, Dr. Paul Dudley White, a prominent advocate of preventive medicine, states that "Healthy exercise is valuable not only for the maintenance of good physiologic function of the body, but also mental clarity, and a feeling of good health." It has long been known that exercise serves as a natural remedy for depression in all ages, in particular regarding how they feel about themselves. Self-concept denotes a set of thoughts held by oneself and about one's self in mental, emotional, and physical realms. Self-esteem refers to the individual's evaluation of his or her self-concept, and self-efficacy is similar to self-confidence in that self-efficacy is a level of certainty that one can perform a task or behavior.

3) Active Isometric (Isotonic)- an active isometric exercise is one that **provides specific movement of a joint or joints off of an isometric holding position**, and does not displace the body over a measurable distance. For example, Hip Rotations, Shoulder Rotations, and Inverted Rotations are examples of Transverse Plane active isometric exercises. These exercises are also focused on correcting misalignment, but also add a strengthening component due to the movement. These exercises use multiple reference points to position the body at right angles to recruit a bilateral engagement or specific joint movement.

4) Dynamic- dynamic exercises actually displace the body over a measurable distance and involve more than one lever. They are designed to strengthen the dynamic muscles to secure an aligned posture. Examples of this would be cross-training, weightlifting, plyometrics, etc.

In summary, the cerebellum, a small part of our lower brain in the back of the head, plays a vital role in coordinating muscles, controlling many reflexes, and keeping us erect in the earth's gravitational field. Recent research demonstrates that the cerebellum's contribution to control of all brain functions — especially cognition and behavior — may be just as great as its control over motor. The cerebellum receives a great portion of its input from the receptors embedded in the joints and muscles. Although humans are not constantly moving, there is a continuous amount of stimulation to the cerebellum from the mechanoreceptors in the joints and muscles, due to the constant load on these structures as a result of gravity. Gravity is thus responsible for providing a source of constant stimuli to our brains. (Azzolino.com)

If the joints and muscles of the body, especially the spinal joints (which receive the majority of the force in the upright posture of humans), are moving correctly, then there is an optimum amount of mechanoreceptor stimulation to the cerebellum and brain, resulting in an appropriate control of the postural muscles. The postural muscles then have increased endurance, allowing them to hold an individual upright for long periods of time.

If an individual has altered biomechanics/movement of a joint, then he may have a decreased amount of mechanoreceptor stimulation to the brain and, in turn, have decreased stimulation to the postural muscles. This could result in a decreased efficiency of these muscles, leading to the question which often arises: What is the best way to improve or maintain postural integrity?

Although exercise of the back muscles is extremely important in this process, many of these back muscles are non-consciously, reflexogenically controlled by the cerebellum; therefore, exercise has a minimal effect. The deepest muscles throughout the spine (together called the intrinsic layer) extend from one vertebra to the next, making them completely dependent on joint motion and reflexive control from the cerebellum. This is why isometric exercises are the most effective in retraining posture because they are most closely associated with the brain.

Another aspect, which I mentioned in the last chapter, was about the ramping factor of a routine. We discussed the amount of time it takes for the average child to get on their feet from birth. The main goal of writing a routine is to progressively ramp a client to the point of standing. With this in mind, we are taking into consideration the number of levers used from start to finish, the goal being to tie the levers as neurologically coordinated as possible so that the brain can understand how to re-pattern one's alignment for a long-term hold. Therefore, the following list of positions from least number of levers to the largest is necessary to understand in order to ramp a routine properly:

1. Lying- the supine position (on your back)
2. Prone-the prone position (on your stomach)
3. Buddha's Pose- a position of sitting on one's heels
4. Hands and Knees
5. Kneeling- a position of one on their knees only
6. Sitting
7. Standing

With these positions in mind it is very important to understand that there is a varied degree of difficulty based on the movement or work being done in each position. Therefore, one must understand the differences between certain positional exercises that will lead to the most appropriate choices for a particular client's needs as we previously discussed. The following pictures describes the basic positions from which all Symmetry corrective postures are derived.

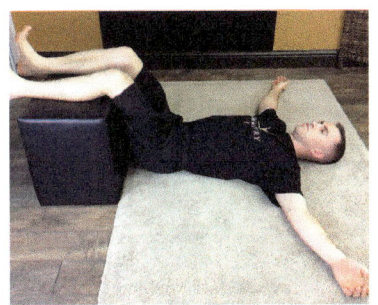
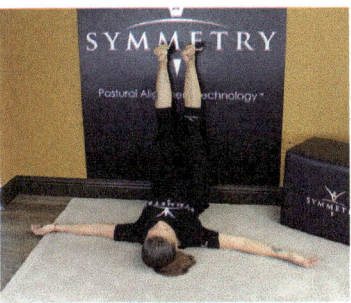
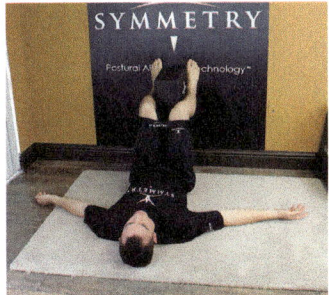

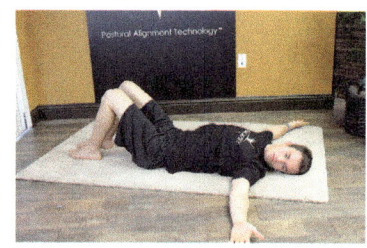 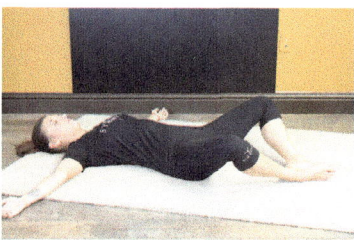 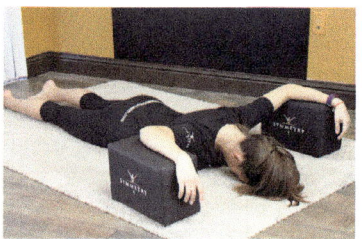
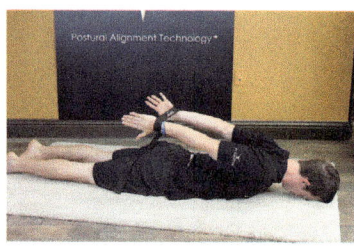 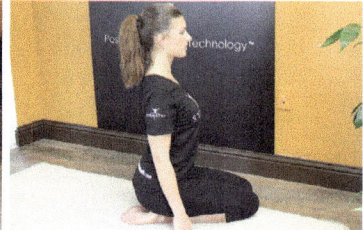 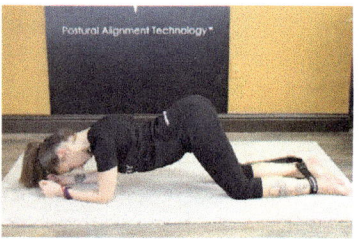
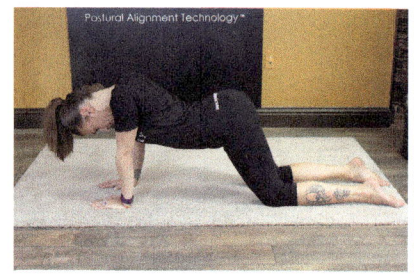 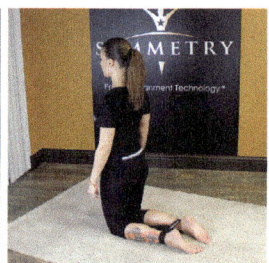 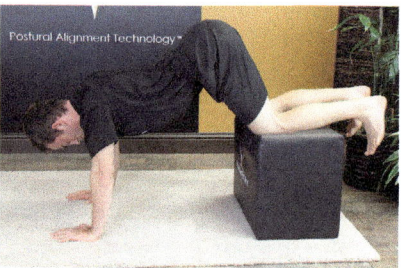
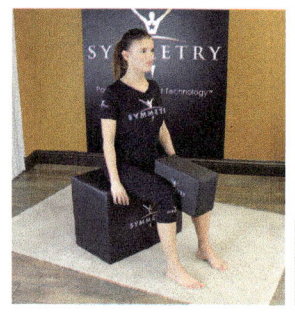 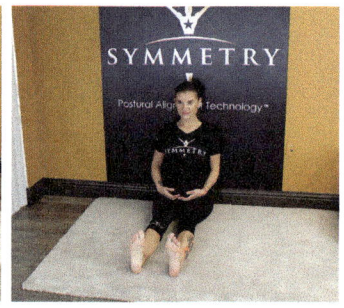 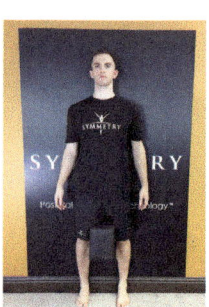

Chapter 12

The AlignSmart™ Technology

In 2007 I was granted a patent for this system. We applied for it in 2003. My advice to you if you are seeking one, start now, and wait impatiently! This system is based on 6 main steps:

1. Label the factors for each client (as stated in the last chapter).
2. Measure the client/you.
3. Generate a report.
4. Create a sequence.
5. Take client/you through the routine.
6. Feel great!

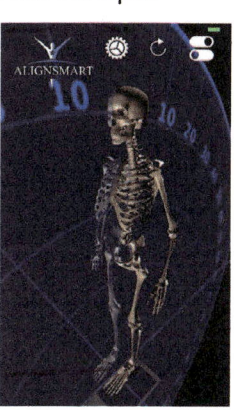

Being that we have already discussed the first two steps, let's talk a lot about step three. It is one thing to assess a client. It is another to quantify a system with measurements. I remember when I was in San Diego, I was able to set up a meeting with the top five Physical Therapists from Sharp Rees Stealy, one of the main medical groups there. As I do with most of my presentations, I asked them if any one of them had any chronic pain. Three out of the five said they did (which again I call "irony") but nonetheless, I targeted one youngster who said he had a chronic shoulder problem. He generously volunteered to be my guinea pig, and I had him take his shirt off. While facing away, I asked the remaining PTs to tell me which shoulder looked elevated. They correctly chose the right, because subjectively, it was way higher than the left. I then took my Palpation Meter, which is what I had at the time, and proceeded to measure the inferior borders of the scapulae, of which it read 7 degrees high on the right side. I then explained that this is an objective way of taking out the "guess work" from typical postural analysis. I then asked them what they thought his pelvis was doing. They looked at me and said, "I'm not sure what you mean?" I then went into my discussion of physics- Newton's third law, and the righting reflex; I explained that the odds were that his left ilium was elevated. I then took my fingers and palpated the crest of his pelvis, of which you could clearly see that his left hip was up. I then measured it, and it read 7 degrees up on the left hip. The question that was then asked was, "How accurate is that device?" They proceeded to critique the system, but I always countered with this question; "What do you measure?" In any case, one of the PTs who was curious in what I had presented, took me to his desk where I showed him my software (albeit the first version). In my discussion with him, I explained to him that regardless of whether they thought my system was inaccurate, theoretically impossible, or just plain stupid, I didn't understand why the PT industry didn't have a similar software program where their patients could report back to them, view their specific rehab exercises, or videos to promote compliance. His answer was very honest. They don't necessarily get paid for clients getting better, just what they can treat, and what insurance will pay for. My wife recently had surgery on her shoulder to clear out some calcium deposits, and after was prescribed Physical Therapy. In the same discussions with the PT, he explained how they had to manipulate the insurance companies due to the fact that they only give them a specific amount of treatments per ailment. And if they want to continue working on the same area, he told my wife that she would have to go back to the doctor for a different diagnosis, then come back to him so that he could continue working on the same area as before. The system doesn't work.

Okay, so, quantifying a system goes beyond just measuring. You have to know how to interpret the measurements, which is what actually makes a system a system. So, how did I come up with the AlignSmart™ system? The one thing that my first programmer told me was that everything in code is actually just mathematical equations or numbers. So, I had to basically write an algorithm that explained the relationships between the planes, the measurements within each plane and the factors associated as numerical values. So, that's what I did. If you take a look at the evaluation sheet again in chapter 10, you will see that the number of measurements in the transverse plane is less than the frontal plane, which is less than the number of measurements in the sagittal plane. Why do you think this is the case? It's because we are primarily sagittal beings as this is the plane we primarily move in. If you look at dynamic training, the majority of movements are linear, or flexion/extension, due to the fact that this is the easiest and most effective way of moving our body from point A to point B. But, alas, I keep talking about structural holding patterns. So, mathematically, if you were to develop a weighted system so that you could quantify the planar relationships, then you would have a way to figure out what disparity is the most important in the process of correcting intrinsic disparities. Let's take most postural assessment programs. They are almost entirely composed of "seeing" the disparity, and not "measuring" the disparity. Again, this is a generic way of evaluating the body, which results in generic treatments. When you place the body in planar categories and then weight them, it becomes very clear as to what needs to be corrected first, and so on. The sequence is the key to success. If you cannot explain objectively why you are treating someone in the sequence you are, then you cannot expect to ever replicate yourself. From this mentality, and after analyzing the planar relationships and weighting them appropriately, I created what I call the Severity-Disparity Chart™. This chart (which is part of the propriety information in our patent), explains exactly how I weighted each measurement within each plane, and then how it relates from plane to plane. Ultimately, this is where a sequence is derived, but for our purposes here, it is important for you to know that if you do not have values assigned in the proper algorithm, then it is impossible to really know where to start your treatment. This is where I always got lost when I was at the Egoscue Method. There was no manuals or equations to guide me to know where to start and where to end. At the end of the day, it was just a series of guesses and hope that a client took to the exercises.

In any case, what I will tell you is that if you look at the ratio between the planes, there is basically a 1:2:3 relationship between the Transverse, Frontal and Sagittal planes and the measurements involved. The transverse plane, being the only horizontal plane, will be the most sensitive to any type of disparity due to the attachments around this plane, and therefore is weighted more heavily in the evaluation process.

It is also the most compensated plane due to this and the fact that most people are one-side dominant, so when they rotate, it is usually to one side primarily, thus promoting over-development of one side. That was me in my 16 years of playing baseball. Depending on the patterns developed over the years and the reasons why, most people come in to our office with large PSIS-ASIS disparities. But guess what? You can't see this measurement! The only way you can understand that there is such a disparity, is if you know what you are looking for, which in most cases is a reaction to this disparity. Pelvic rotation, an elevated ilium, knee rotation, spinal offsets, are all results of a PSIS-ASIS disparity, but at the end of the day, even if you do know what you are looking for, you don't know to what degree the disparity is, and if it needs to be addressed initially or not. What I do know, is that therapies do not measure this and make the mistake of treating what I call the by-product result, which is usually the site of pain. In our system, I can tell you that almost all clients who come in initially are more despaired in the transverse plane, which should be addressed initially before anything else. In my humble opinion, the mistake that most therapies make is addressing a patient's issues with sagittal plane exercises first. Let me give you an example. I had a client come in the other day, post knee surgery as a result of wear and tear, a non-contact injury. He had gone through 3 months of physical therapy, and when I measured him, I explained to him that his opposite hip was the problem. He looked at me funny, because to him, his knee still hurt, not his opposite hip, so that must be the problem. As I reviewed his report I explained that his opposite hip was so posterior that it was causing his other hip to take on most of the compensation, leading to his knee to externally rotate on the same side- the side he had surgery on. You see, you can't just simply treat an area of pain without understanding where it is coming from. And this is how traditional therapy works. Most knee rehab is done in the sagittal plane- flexion extension. However, if the problem originates from the PSIS-ASIS, then this has to be corrected with rotational exercises first before you can even think about rehabbing the knee. So, the sequence matters. It matters a lot, because if you are treating the body in the wrong order, then the default pattern of compensation will always win. This is also why adjustments rarely hold. But with a properly sequenced routine, in conjunction with any treatment, the body will recover faster than you can imagine!

So, let's talk about the system itself. The following steps explain how the system works for both the practitioner's and client's perspective:

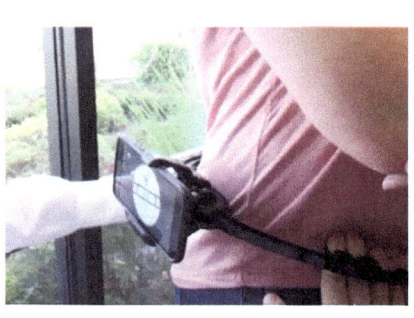

1. The practitioner or client logs in on their mobile device or tablet once they have downloaded the AlignSmart™ App on their device.

2. The practitioner then clicks on "New Evaluation" for specific client. The client will click on "My Dashboard" to access their routines, reports, photos, etc.

3. The practitioner then takes all of the measurements and voice-commands them into our AlignSmart™ Bluetooth system.

4. Once the measurements are completed, a report is generated, which quantifies the evaluation,

and is the main tool of education for the client. The scale ranges from "0" (meaning perfectly aligned) to "27" (meaning very misaligned) for each plane, and the overall range is from 0-81 points. This is like, golf, you want a low score!

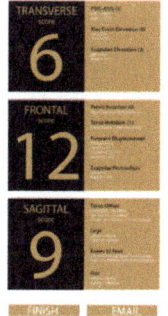

5. Depending on your level of cerification, the practitioner can manipulate the app. For a "Level 4" practitioner, they have the ability to evaluate the client and generate a report. From there they can print the report out, or email it to the client for their records. This way it can be monitored from session to session. A "Level 5" practitioner can evaluate their client, generate a report AND a unique sequence of exercises that the client can then perform on a daily basis. This level however, the

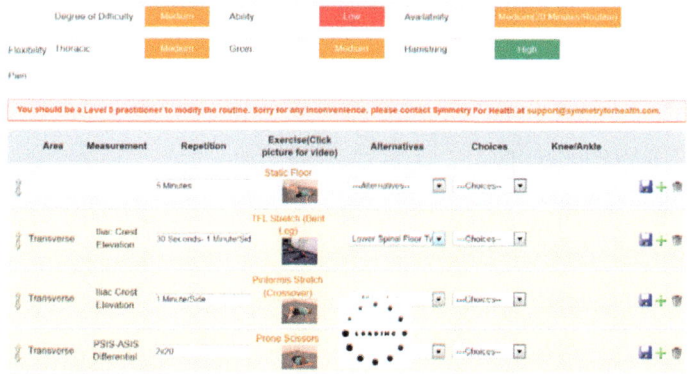

practitioner cannot manipulate the suggested routine by the software. So, the choices that the software will suggest will tend to be more on the conservative side and is used mainly to help support the main treatment model of the practitioner.

6. A "Level 6" practitioner can do all of the above AND have final editing power over the software, which means that due to the extensive knowledge the practitioner has

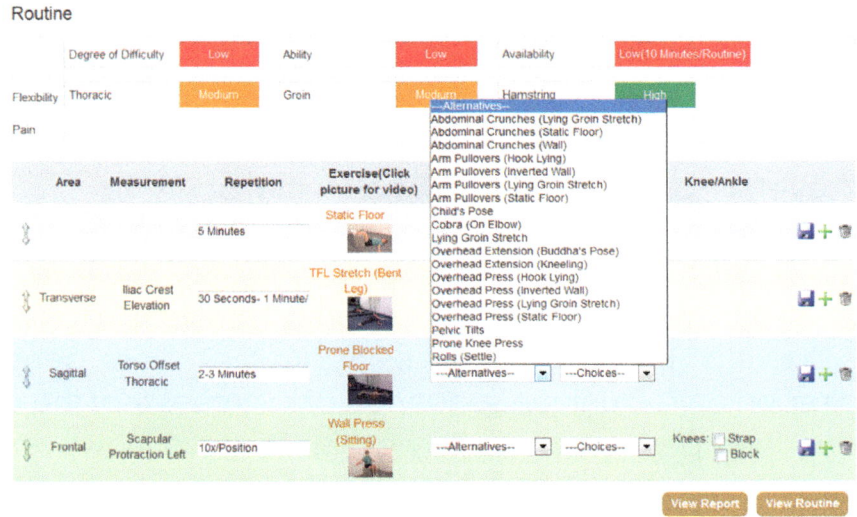

of their clients, they can "fine-tune" the routine if necessary, which gives the practitioner ultimate control over their client's well-being.

Once the practitioner completes the edits, they can then take their patient/client through the routine, and/or send them a text for the client to then log in on their AligSmart™ app and watch the videos in the sequence they are given, and then begin to perform the routine regularily at home until the next session. Again, this is where this system thrives because we are changing the game. The main emphasis of this program is to make sure the client is a proactive participant in their

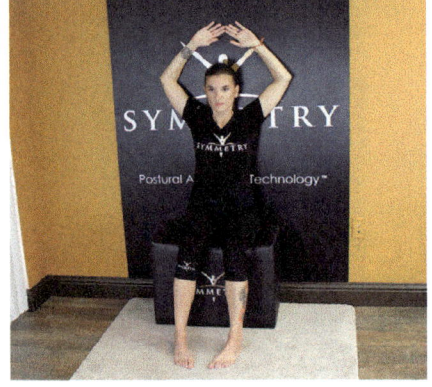

healing and health process. All other treatments become the tools to help this process along, mainly because you can only treat people so many times a week. With this sytem, if educated properly, clients will do their routines twice a day for a 3- month period. And we have proven that they will do this. This encompasses nearly 200 opportunities for a client to perform their specific sequenced routines. We actually educate them to treat each routine attempt as a "treatment" session. They are just taking their treatment home with them, because they can. But, we check in with them, and they check in with us to keep the responsibility a two-way street. However, we ask them if they were to pay for any treatment for a total of 200 times, how much would that cost them? Let's say at an average of $50 per session, this would be a $10,000 investment, which by the way, Forbes.com confirmed that this is the amount that the average person now pays per year on health care. Crazy!!!

If you want to toy around with our Level 1 AlignSmart app right now, go to your "store" on your phone, search for "AlignSmart" and download if for free. You can manually manipulate the entire skeleton by swiping your finger across the screen, and if you click on the buttons on the top right, you will see a list of areas that you can specifically manipulate. For level 1, you only get to play with the PSIS-ASIS angles and the Spinal Offset. The rest are locked 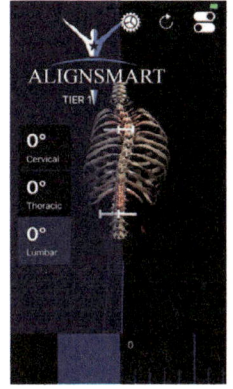 unless you upgrade to Level 2 or higher. But this is a fun way of checking out what your skeleton looks like in 3-D! Your kids will love it!

Chapter 13

Try it out for Yourself!

Okay. Hopefully you have been intrigued thus far to want to delve a little deeper. This is where the "self-help" portion of the book comes in that I swore I would never do again like my first book. You see, the problem with self-help books is that they have to be generically written to a broad audience and hope that whatever is suggested for you to do will somehow stick and make you feel amazing! It is IMPOSSIBLE for any expert to write a book, sell you on a philosophy, and then give you the magic potion in a book. Even if you have success with these different types of books, and I can give you a list, I guarantee it will be short-lived. Why? Let me explain. There are 12 systems that run the human body:

1. The circulatory system
2. The digestive system
3. The endocrine system
4. The immune system
5. The lymphatic system
6. The nervous system
7. The muscular system

8. The reproductive system

9. The skeletal system

10. The respiratory system

11. The urinary system

12. The integumentary system

The human body contains over 100 trillion cells. The human brain contains about 100 billion nerve cells. In the skeletal and muscular system alone, there are 856 parts that run these systems, and thousands of parts for the remaining systems. Why do I give you this information? Because there are so many variables to the human body that it is impossible to understand you, the reader, to the extent that I would confidently know how to treat you with this book! So, am I an expert in my field? I suppose some would argue this, but I am not about to tell you that if you perform the following example routines, you will be cured of your ailments. Yes, to check off my box, consult with your doctor first. HOWEVER, I will tell you that in my 21 years in this field, I can confidently give you a couple of choices of corrective sequences that fall within the general margins of what most people present to me when they first come in. With that being said, to again paint you a clearer picture, the average client comes in for at least three months in our program, assessed six times during this time-frame and given a unique sequence each time based upon the system I have already mentioned. It takes at least three months for the body to start showing consistent holding patterns, and then three months of strengthening to make sure it holds. THEN, we educate our clients on how to maintain this. Why do I tell you this? Because it is 1% of 1% of the population that is motivated enough to even take a system presented in a book and actually complete the entire process presented in such a book. So, experience the following routines with the understanding that this is just a taste of how to get the body to start releasing your years of compensation patterns and touch on the strengthening process. What you will more than likely feel with the first routine is a very positive result right away. This is mainly due to unwinding the transverse issues that most people show, so the tension caused by this pattern will usually give you immediate relief. Do this routine for at least one to two weeks, twice a day if you are motivated, and then switch to the second one. The second routine you will not feel as great as you did with the first one. This is due to the fact that most of your large disparities will be corrected in the first routine, which gives you the most unwinding, which results in the most relief. But, it will be temporary as your body then adjusts as the new layers of dysfunction rear their ugly head. Our recommendation after this is to either find an AlignSmart™ specialist near you to complete the entire process, or take the two routines and rotate between them on a semi-weekly basis. This will at least keep you in somewhat control over your issues and allow for you to have some consistent correction to rely on every day. But, it won't take you to the promised land. Nothing ever great in life is easy to achieve. You have just been conditioned to rely on the "experts" so that you can't ever really get better and also so that you keep contributing your hard-earned dollars to the pit of recycled wellness. It's capitalism at its best!

If you run into an exercise or two that are either contradicted by your doctor's advice, or you just don't feel good while doing it, either skip the exercise or give an AlignSmart specialist a call to help you out. We have 350 corrective exercises to choose from if you were to go through the entire program, so we can certainly help you out with suggesting an alternative exercise. However, please make sure that you are performing the routines in the sequence they were given. It does make a difference. (Please email us at info@symmetryforhealth.com if you would like access to the video links to these routines)

ROUTINE #1:

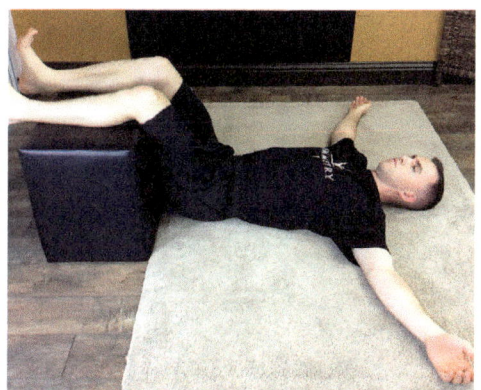

Static Floor: Lie on your back with both legs on an 18-20-inch block, knees bent to 90 degrees. Keep your arms out to your side with your palms up. Relax your back into the floor and breathe through your diaphragm. Stay in this position for **5 minutes**.

Hip Rotations (Static Floor): Lying on your back with your knees and hips bent at 90 degrees and legs on an 18-inch block or chair, place your feet together with your toes pulled back half way out on the block. KEEPING YOUR

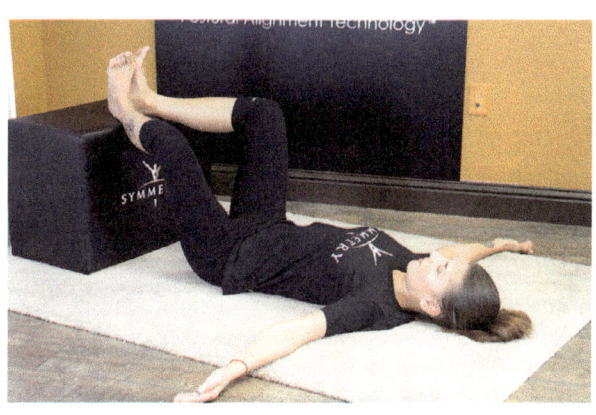

FEET STRAIGHT AND TOGETHER slowly spread your knees apart while pivoting on the inside of your feet as they stay together. Do not let your feet separate as your knees widen apart and try to keep them flexed throughout the motion.

Your practitioner may have you place a 6-inch block in between your feet for more support. **Perform 2 sets of 10 to 20 repetitions.**

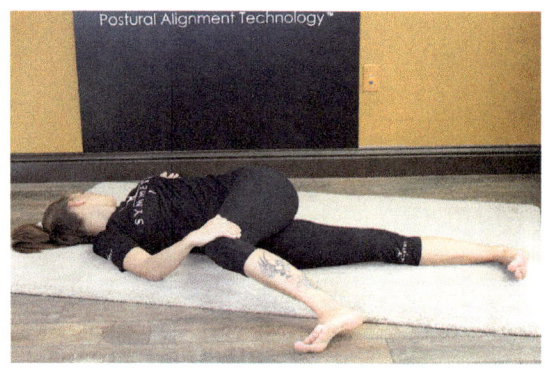

TFL Stretch (Bent Leg): Start on your back with your legs straight out, knees and feet hip-width and pointing up to the ceiling. Keep your arms straight out from your side with your palms up. Tighten one leg and flex your foot back, raise the other leg to 90 degrees at the hip and then bend that knee to 90 degrees. Take your opposite hand and reach to the outside of the elevated knee and pull your entire leg across your body without the opposite shoulder rising off the floor. Make sure that your other leg stays tight, feet flexed at the ankle. Look the opposite direction and keep your stomach and upper torso RELAXED. BREATHE! Hold for the allotted amount of time and then switch. **Hold for 30 seconds to 1 minute per side.**

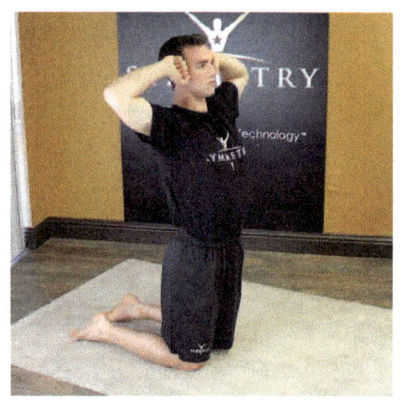

Shoulder Rotations (Kneeling): Kneeling, induce an arch in your lower back by rolling your hips forward and not by leaning your torso back. Position your hands with your knuckles on your temples, palms facing to the front. Keeping your knuckles on your temples and your wrists from bending, bring your elbows together and touch in front of your chest, but chin-high, with your palms now facing each other. Try to keep your head still by not bobbing it back and forth as you try and touch your elbows together. Then separate your elbows by pulling your arms back, squeezing your shoulder blades together and then repeat. Keep your stomach relaxed by inhaling as you separate your elbows and exhaling as you bring your elbows together. **Perform 2 sets of 10 to 20 repetitions.**

Extended Ankle Abduction: Start with your hands and knees hip-width and perpendicular to floor. Walk your hands forward 4-6 inches and allow your shoulders to reposition over your hands without moving your knees on the floor. With your hips now in front of your 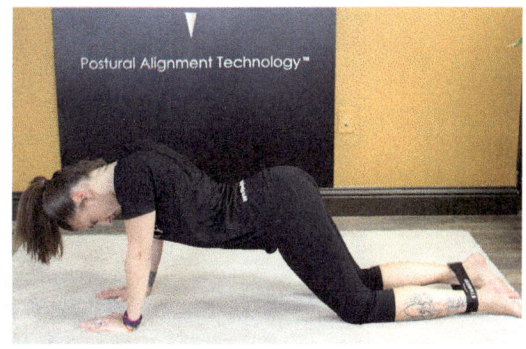 knees, allow your back to sway, shoulder blades to collapse together, and head to drop, but keep your elbows locked. While holding this position, press out on a strap hip-width at your ankles for one second and then release. Feel the contraction on the outside of your hips. Breathe and relax stomach. In between each set, keep your hands in the same position and push your body back to stretch out your lower back. **Perform 2 sets of 10 to 20 repetitions.**

Hip Adduction (Sitting): Sitting with your knees bent to 90

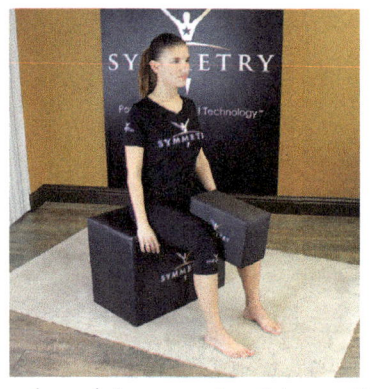

degrees, place a 6-inch block between your knees. With your feet straight, arms to your side, press in against the block and release for one second, relaxing your stomach and shoulders. Exhale as you press in and inhale as you relax. Allow your back to be slightly arched by rolling your pelvis forward and your shoulders pulled together without shrugging. **Perform 2 sets of 10 to 20 repetitions.**

ROUTINE #2:

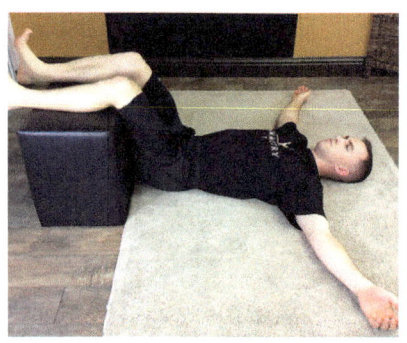

Static Floor: Lie on your back with both legs on an 18-20 -inch block, knees bent to 90 degrees. Keep your arms out to your side with your palms up. Relax your back into the floor and breathe through your diaphragm. Stay in this position for **5 minutes**.

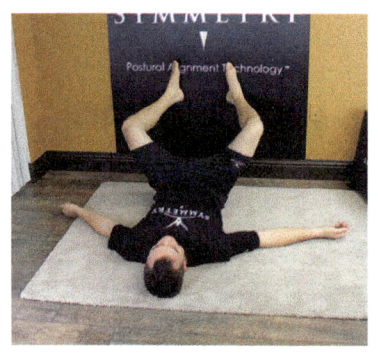

Hip Rotations (Wall): Lying on your back with your knees and hips bent at 90 degrees, place your feet hip-width and straight on a wall. KEEPING YOUR FEET STRAIGHT (Almost pigeon-toed) slowly spread your knees apart while pivoting on the outside of your feet keeping your heels on the wall, then bring your knees together and then repeat. After each set, reposition your feet correctly on the wall if necessary. Keep your stomach relaxed and rest in between each set for a duration of two deep breaths. **Perform 2 sets of 10 to 20 repetitions.**

Piriformis Stretch (Crossover): Lie on your back with your knees bent, feet on the floor, and hip-width. Cross your left ankle to right knee and pivot off the outside of your right foot and rotate your left foot and right knee to the floor as 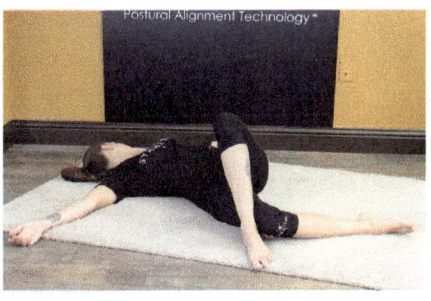 one unit. Make sure to not let your right foot slide in as you rotate on its side. Keeping your left foot flat on floor, press your left knee slightly away feeling a stretch on the outside of the left hip. Place arms out to side, relax your shoulders and stomach and look the opposite direction. **Hold for 30 seconds to 1 minute per side.**

Arm Glides (Inverted Wall): Lie on your back with legs straight up on a wall, feet hip-width apart. With your quads tight position your body away from wall, if necessary, so that your tailbone and back rests on the floor. Keeping your knees pointed straight off the wall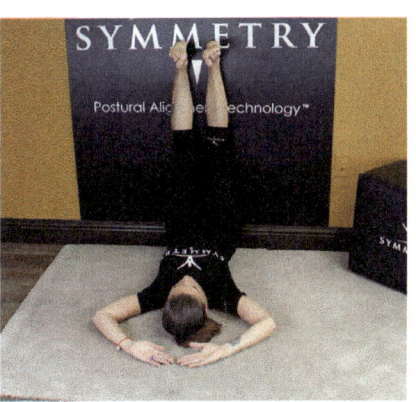

and toes flexed back, feel a stretch in hamstrings and calves. Keep your feet flat as if you were trying to hold a drink on them. Relax your stomach and hold this position. Proceed to bend your elbows at 90-degrees placing your arms and back of hands on the floor. Maintaining a 90-degree angle, slowly raise your arms overhead until your hands touch. Keep your elbows, forearms and hands slightly pressed into floor. Return to starting position and repeat for allotted number of repetitions. Be sure to inhale and allow your back to arch as you reach arms overhead. As this first position becomes easier, glide arms higher by touching hands further above your head. Relax in between each set and rest for the duration of two deep breaths. **Perform 2 sets of 10 repetitions.**

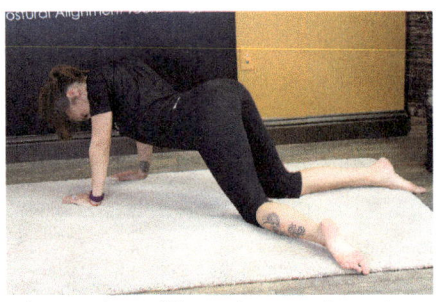

Hip Rotations (Extended Floor Position): Start with your hands and knees hip-width and perpendicular to the floor. Walk your hands forward 4-6 inches and allow your shoulders to reposition over your hands without moving knees on floor. Let your back sway with shoulder blades together and arms straight. Proceed to slide your feet apart while staying in contact with the floor, pivoting off of your knees, feeling the rotation from your hip joint. Separate your feet as much as you can, feeling the stretch in your hips, then bring your feet back together and repeat, keeping your form throughout the exercise. In between sets, push your butt back to your heels to stretch out your back for a few seconds, then repeat. **Perform 2 sets of 10 to 20 repetitions.**

Hip Abduction (Static): Sitting tall by rolling your pelvis forward with your knees bent to 90 degrees, place a strap around your knees either together or hip-width. With your feet straight, arms to your side, press out against the strap and HOLD for the recommended amount of time, relaxing your stomach and shoulders. Breathe. **Hold for 1 to 2 minutes.**

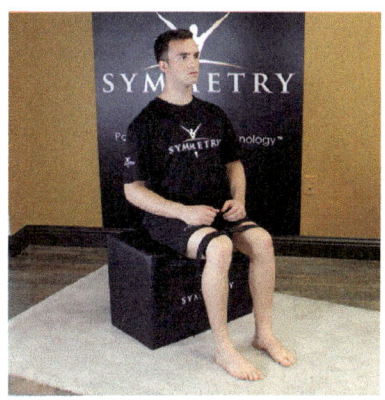

Wall Sit: With your low back against a wall, slowly walk your feet away from the wall. Keeping your feet hip-width apart and straight ahead, slide down the wall until your knees are at 90-degree angle or just above. Press your low back into the wall by placing the weight on your heels and not your toes. Keep your stomach and shoulders relaxed. Feel in your thighs. You may be advised to place a block or a strap at your knees for further support. **Hold for 1 to 2 minutes.**

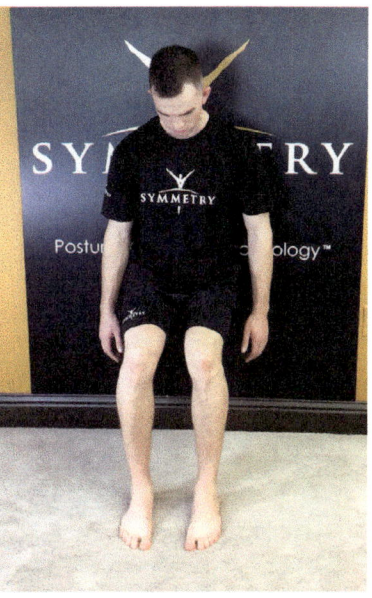

Chapter 14

Success!

I have been blessed with the path that I have been fortunate enough to travel. It has indeed been the one less traveled, but I would have never experienced what I have experience if I had gone the traditional route. It has definitely been the riskier route as well, but with great risk comes great reward. Every day I get to interact with people who have been sullied by the system, and left with dismal choices. When I see my clients progressing to long-term wellness, it is the greatest joy on the planet to hear them explain how it feels to be out of pain, and that they realize that they did it themselves. I get thanked every day, but the reality, and what I tell them, is that they did all the hard work. We just bossed them around, with lots of love and motivation, of course.

Our mission now is to certify every willing practitioner out there who believes that we as practitioners are just the conduit to teaching people how to become well again. What I love about the AlignSmart™ system is that it provides the tools and education for people who are tired of being sick and tired, the real opportunity to becoming healthy again, reaching goals they once thought were impossible. I live this every day myself. My love now is playing basketball. Every time I play, I spend most of the time doing my routine before I play, because I know what I know. I have been playing at my gym now for 9 years, and knock on wood, I have avoided serious injury because I prepare myself daily and have no fear anymore of pushing my body to its limits. Most everyone else shows up, grabs a ball, and starts shooting. And if they do stretch, it's the same thing each time. They just don't know what they don't know. I want to educate the world as to why this system should be the main source of wellness, in all models. If you don't know what to do and why to do it on a daily basis, then at the end of the day you too are just guessing as to how to become well again.

The following testimonials are from some of my favorite clients. They indeed are the reason we do what we do. Enjoy!

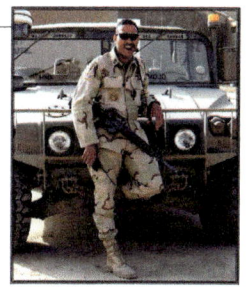

"I am a 42-year-old veteran of the United States Army, of which I spent 22 years in active duty. In that time, I worked as a paratrooper-mechanic, infantryman and drill instructor. The activities I participated in on a daily basis include but were not limited to 4 to 10 mile runs in the morning with calisthenics; 4, 8 and 12 mile foot marches with 60 pound rucksack, heavy lifting in every conceivable position on a daily basis, airborne operations with combat equipment exceeding 265 pounds and the ever faithful standard of putting your weapon into operation once you land, recover your equipment and double-time it to the assembly area with all that equipment on your person. Hopefully one could find it in the darkness in a reasonable amount of time. What is the bottom line? You had to be mentally and physically tough to endure these rigors.

After 22 years of training troops and doing Uncle Sam's business abroad, I retired a back-broken individual who woke daily to sharp pains which ran up my back and down the back of my legs. In x-rays, my L-4 and 5 were black! I thought I would need surgery and spend the rest of my life taking medication. Little did I know that my life would take a drastic change for the better in December of 2006. The first time I was told about Symmetry by Patrick Mummy, I was skeptical. If there were such a solution for my back pain, the military would be an intricate and developmental part of it. After all, I served honorably and deserve the best! After getting measured and going through my first routine, I will admit I felt better. However, I was still very skeptical that exercises would alleviate my pain. I was given a Symmetry routine and continued to follow that routine's guidelines until I finished. Then I went on to my second routine and then third. I have not felt this limber and agile since I was a young paratrooper in the 82nd Airborne Division. It is just amazing!

I can tell you quite honestly that I quit doing the routine once. But that lasted all of 10 days, until my back pain became so unbearable that I had to restart my routine. Two days after restarting, the pain was totally gone. Why do I sing the unsolicited praises of something I have to pay for? Because it works and I think everyone who experiences back pain should learn of this program and do it to improve their standard of living. Back pain can be stressful, and today, I am stress free!" Thank you, Patrick, and Symmetry!"

Joseph A. Thomas, Master Sergeant, United States Army (Retired)

Symmetry – The Best Thing I've Ever Won

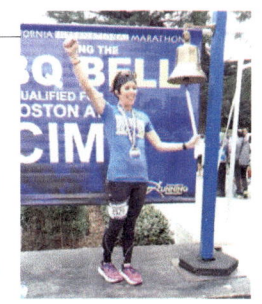

"When it comes to raffle prizes or drawings, I never win. I just don't. In the spring of 2014, my luck changed at a charity golf tournament. I threw some tickets into a basket for this item called "Symmetry, Postural Alignment Technology™" because it looked interesting. The next thing I knew, they were calling MY number! I won! At the time, I didn't care that it was for Symmetry, I was just happy to finally win!

After the thrill of victory passed, my Symmetry package sat in an envelope on my desk at home for a few months. One day while cleaning, I found it and decided to call and make an appointment. I'm always a little skeptical about new approaches to health and wellness. And, as a busy wife, mother and business owner, finding time to do something like this is always problematic. But this package was worth over $1,000, so I thought I might as well check it out. One phone call and a week later, I walked into the place that would turn my current perspective of my structural wellbeing upside down.

The first thing I discovered is Symmetry is a happy place; like the kind of happy you find among good friends. Seriously. Upon entering a pleasantly decorated office with big windows, I was greeted by the larger-than-life enthusiasm of Symmetry founder, Patrick Mummy, and his equally friendly colleague, Phaedra Jackson. After approaching me like they've known me for years and offering me tea, we proceeded to chat. They asked me a series of questions about my health concerns, exercise habits and physical pain level. They explained the theory behind

Symmetry and how having our bodies in alignment eliminates a lot of physical health problems and chronic pain issues. Patrick then pulled out this funky little measuring device he developed called a Postural Alignment Tool, which measures specific misalignments. Still skeptical, I listened. He went on to tell me about how this device works and how I would be able to correct my misalignment with exercise routines I would do at home. It made sense and sounded easy enough, but did it work, and did I need it?

Then it began...the measuring, the evaluation, and the truth about my personal symmetry situation. Patrick and Phaedra measured my alignment and entered my numbers into Symmetry's patented software program. This software calculates your measurements three-dimensionally to determine postural issues and the specific exercises needed to correct each one. As they were taking measurements of my spine, hips and shoulders, and evaluating the placement of my knees, feet and head, I kept thinking, "How bad can I be? I can't be that out of line, can I?" After it was all over, I was about to enter the first phase of the Symmetry school of humility. What's worse, they had the photos to prove it. In addition to the numbers revealed by the software, they also take a few photos of you in front of a grid so they can visually point out to you where you are misaligned. It's important to note they do all this evaluating with you fully dressed; perfect for modest gals like me.

It's a good thing I was sitting down when the software kicked out alignment numbers and they showed me the photos. I was a misaligned, lopsided, forward-tilting, knock-kneed mess. On a scale of 0 to 27 with 0 being perfect alignment, I scored a 24 in the Transverse category (elevation of hips, shoulders); an 11 in the Frontal category (body rotation); and 15 in the Sagittal category (offset of spine, head, shoulders, knees, feet) for a total score of 50. Yikes! What's worse, Patrick knew exactly what I was experiencing from a pain and physical symptoms standpoint without me having to tell them. I was like an open book – I had been officially busted.

After swallowing my pride and conceding the fact that I had some serious alignment problems, they proceeded to devise my first exercise routine. The Symmetry exercise routine is based on two things: 1) where you need correction and 2) how much time you have each day to commit to the routine. Based on my input, Patrick created a 15-minute routine that I was to complete twice daily. To make sure you do everything correctly, you receive the exercises on paper, do the routine under a watchful eye at the office, and if you still have questions, you can watch video demonstrations online. Patrick's background is in physical technology, so the exercises reflect his knowledge of the human musculoskeletal system and are directly connected to a multitude of symptoms exposed in the evaluation.

Enter the second phase of the Symmetry school of humility. Exercises that looked easy on paper quickly brought me to my knees (literally) when I had to lie on the floor and contort myself into all sorts of ridiculous positions. This was only made more challenging by repetitive motions that worked various parts of my body into exhaustion; "feel the burn" type of exhaustion. I have been physically fit my entire life, so why was this so hard and awkward? All the while, Patrick and Phaedra smiled with one of those "We told her so!" type grins that made me want to prove to them that I really could do this. As I got in my car to drive home, I decided I'd give it a few weeks and see for myself if this Symmetry thing was the real deal.

Two weeks later, I returned for my first evaluation. I quickly got the tangible proof I needed in my sore body and my next set of numbers. My total score plummeted from a 50 to a 30. The process of breaking years of alignment issues from sitting at work, playing sports, carrying toddlers on my hip, lifting heavy objects, and who knows what else, was happening. My body was willing to correct itself, but I had to be willing to make the commitment to continue. For the next two months, I went to Symmetry every two weeks for a check-up. Each time I went back, I would get measured, we'd discuss symptoms, and I would come home with a new set of exercises. Unfortunately, the exercises did not get easier nor did finding the time to do them. But discipline is the main reason Symmetry works. If you don't do the work, you can't make the corrections.

As I write this, after I began what I like to call the raffle-winning Symmetry experiment, I am now in the maintenance phase. My numbers are now 3 (Transverse), 5 (Frontal) and 3 (Sagittal) for a total score of 11, which if you don't know what this means- it's great! What am I feeling? I am feeling a lot less pain (I have Fibromyalgia), my hips don't make a "popping" noise any more, my knees aren't so turned in, my spine is straight, and when I run, my body feels 10 years younger. Do I still feel some soreness with my exercises? Yes. My body is still correcting itself and I'm okay with that. I feel a sense of accomplishment knowing that I am taking charge of my physical health with non-invasive technology that is helping me now AND preventing issues down the road. Feeling good today is nice, but knowing I can prevent hip surgery, pain medication, and back issues down the road is even better. Even though Symmetry's exercises are hard and make me look ridiculous, I'll take it!

Having my body in alignment has improved my speed and recovery for distance running. Any runner will tell you that as you pile on the miles training for a race, you run the risk of some type of injury. I have become so much stronger due to Symmetry that I decided to increase the intensity of my training in an attempt to qualify for the Boston Marathon. What I once thought was impossible became a reality! On December 4, 2016, I ran a Boston Qualifying (BQ) time of 3:36:13. And it doesn't end there. In February of 2017, I ran my first ultra marathon on a trail, a 50k distance (31 miles), and finished 47th out of more than 250 runners. And I could walk the next day! Simply put, Symmetry is the platform that enables your body to achieve its potential. You must have alignment coincide with training and diet to be at your best.

Do I now understand why Symmetry is such a happy place and why Patrick and his associates are so excited about their jobs? Absolutely. What Patrick has created in Symmetry is a pathway to better structural and physical health for the long-term. He challenges the traditional paradigm of the quick fix, over-medicating and fad solutions. Symmetry is not about being temporary; it's about lasting change and empowerment to feel and look better. If you are seeking a real difference in your wellness, don't hesitate to put your tickets in the Symmetry basket. You might just discover you won the lottery."

Mary Anne Copley

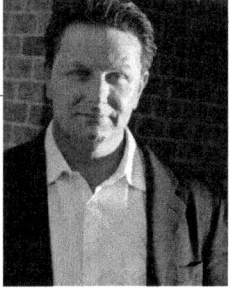

"As a recipient of the Symmetry AlignSmart™ system, I have been able to make adjustments to my body and sustain my level of activity in the gym 4 to 5 times a week as well as increase my performance on the Golf course. Most importantly, I have been able to increase the quality of my life by being able to put my body in the optimal position in gravity, thus allowing gravity to be my friend and not foe.

As a 23-year practicing Holistic Health practitioner / certified structural integrative therapist / injury treatment specialist, I have seen the efficacy of my treatments increase by upwards of 50% thus increasing my client base the same 50 %. Adding the Symmetry AlignSmart™ programming and the measurements to show exactly what posture / strength / stretching components plus the ability to do comparison analysis pre/post, is invaluable. Without question, this should be a modality in every form of P.T and technology in my opinion."

Kelley Schlager, HHP, Certified structural integrationist/Rolfer, CHEK practitioner, Certified AlignSmart™ Specialist

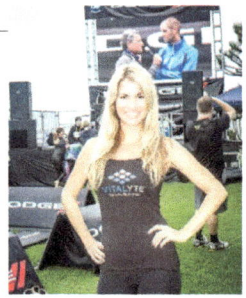

"Throughout my professional running career, I won multiple national titles and was ranked amongst the finest runners in the world. Once I retired I knew I needed to tend to my body so I could have a good quality of life, post-athletics. Symmetry has been a big part of the "wellness" recipe I follow. Now, at the age of 41, I feel better than ever. And when I have women half my age ask me how I stay in such great shape, I know I'm doing something right!"

Milena Glusac
7 time NCAA All American
3 time US National Champion
Top 10 finisher at Boston and New York Marathon

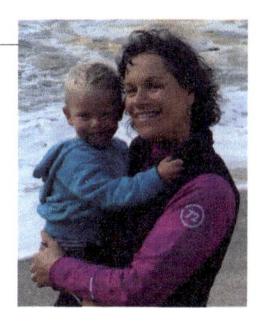

"I was in my mid-forties, swimming with the Masters team and doing hot yoga when old injuries came back to haunt me. My right shoulder was grinding during swim workouts and increasing pain in my right hip was resulting in a limp. How could I maintain a healthy active lifestyle if I couldn't walk and couldn't swim without pain? A medical doctor who had been helped by Patrick referred me to Symmetry. Today I am pain-free and have flexibility, which is a good thing because I have to keep up with my 7 kids. Since the chronic pain is behind me, I have been able to move more and have lost weight. I love being in control of my treatment by doing my routine regularly. I am no longer tied to the chiropractor's office. Everyone that I have referred to Symmetry has experienced sweet relief, including my very skeptical, inactive, MD husband. It works!"

Lesley Lidge

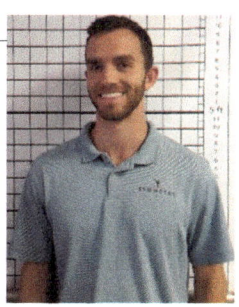

"I discovered Symmetry in the spring of 2015 in a time of pure desperation. I had chronic patellar pain in both knees, on and off sciatica in my left hip, pain in my right upper back, and tendonitis in both forearms. During this time, I was a personal trainer at a sports club and a strength coach for a boys' gymnastics team, and although I had a reputation for being obsessed with rehabilitation and posture, it was my own body that was constantly falling apart! In addition to this, I had a Bachelor's Degree in Exercise Science and was looking to start Physical Technology school in the fall. But for all my investment in continued education, internships, research, and work experience, I couldn't get my own body out of pain. The system from which I was learning, was missing something critical.

I was so desperate for relief that I even started writing my own book, a compilation of my experiences and knowledge regarding rehabilitation of chronic injuries. Not surprisingly, the realization that I came to during this process was that postural dysfunction causes muscular compensation patterns to form throughout the body, which in turn causes inefficient movement, thus damage to the joints.

Around this time, I was introduced to Patrick by one of the gymnastics coaches I worked with. My first thought was: "It's too simple! These exercises are too easy to make lasting postural changes…" But after some time of doing my Symmetry routine, and examining the logic behind the measurement and sequencing process, I had to admit: Patrick was about 20 years ahead of me on the same journey I was so strongly set upon. And he understood my struggle from the very start! The fact that he experienced the same shortcomings of our healthcare system, and created Symmetry out of necessity to heal his own injuries remains one of my greatest inspirations.

Fast forward to Fall of 2016: I am a Postural Therapist working for Symmetry at the main office in Folsom; right where my journey began, but I'm definitely not the same person I used to be! I have been out of chronic pain for over a year. Since starting work with Symmetry I have seen and helped hundreds of individuals who, just like myself, were out of options and looking for a last ditch effort to get their lives back on track.

Symmetry for me represents so much more than just posture and pain relief: It is a symbol of not giving up. It is a symbol of the relentless pursuit of the scientific method, the determination to not settle for mediocre or incomplete results that are "just good enough," but to go above and beyond to find out the innermost causes of a problem so it can be addressed effectively.

Thank you, Patrick Mummy, for never giving up."

Andrew "AJ" Juntunen, B.S. Exercise Science, CSCS, SPP

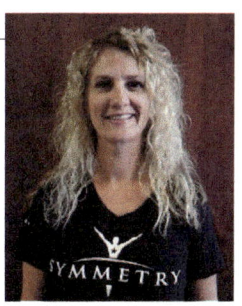

"I was a ballet dancer and in pain since the age of 12 and diagnosed with Scoliosis. Nothing I tried helped my pain so I just learned to live with it. I became a Certified Massage Therapist wanting to help others when I couldn't help myself. After 10 years, I was physically exhausted and in more pain after giving multiple massages every day. I found Symmetry in 2014 and this process has changed my life! Symmetry made such an impact on me that I have changed careers and am now a certified AlignSmart™ therapist. I wish I would have known about Symmetry when I was a massage therapist because I would have referred all my clients to Symmetry to help them rid themselves of pain permanently. I am no longer in pain nor have Scoliosis and I also lost a significant amount of weight. My outlook and quality of life has completely changed and I love living pain free!"

Lee Anne Carson, CMT, Certified AlignSmart™ Specialist

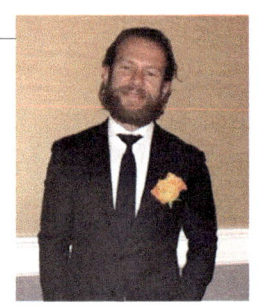

"My name is Andy Rocklin and I discovered Symmetry for Health back in 2011. Throughout my life, I have always been an active person who played many sports, including competitive soccer. In 1997 and 1998 I had two knee surgeries that replaced my meniscus and fixed my MCL and ACL. And since those two surgeries, I had recurring issues in one of my knees, thus causing one to be weaker than the other. My knee would hurt, I would pull muscles and experience chronic lower back tightness. My doctor, who was doing her best to help me with my ongoing issues, recommended that I see Patrick Mummy, as he specializes in fixing ailments like my own. So, I visited the Symmetry office and on my first evaluation I scored a 68, which is not very good at all! He explained how his system works and why I was constantly hurting in one area or the other. Being a highly-motivated person, I like the fact that the treatment was in my own hands and that I can do the exercises on my own time, as often as I could and therefore help myself get better. I think it's one of the best parts about the system, that the patient helps themselves. Symmetry routines can be done anywhere and anytime. So, I went thought the program and started feeling much better. I was and still am injury free for over 5 years now.

But that's not the end of the story… During one of the sessions with Patrick, he told me that not only does he treat people that are hurting, but that he also teaches his system to practitioners, so that they can help others get better. This was very inspiring to me and due to the nature of my work and interests, I inquired as to how successful this second part of his business. I was expecting to hear that he had trained thousands of practitioners and that this system is healing people all over the world. I was very surprised to hear a much smaller number, and so I offered Patrick my help and knowledge to take this out into the world so that thousands of people could get help and benefit from this amazing system. That is when the partnership was born and grew from there. Fast forward five years and we are finally on the verge of re-introducing this technology to the world. Our goal is to train Symmetry practitioners all over the world to help as many people as possible enjoy a pain-free, healthy lifestyle. I can't say enough about how amazing Patrick and what he created is. I have seen many walk away from pain, cancel their surgeries and enjoy an overall better quality of life."

Andy Rocklin, Entrepreneur

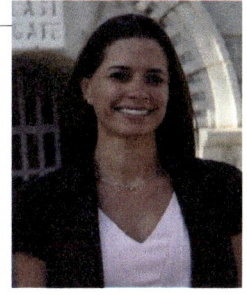

"I am grateful I gave Symmetry a try. I have a very active life and love my various workouts. I started walking with a "hitch" as I put it and began getting really bad hip pain. After trying standard pain relief options, I reluctantly got a Cortisone shot. That only took away the shooting pain I had going down my leg but the hip pain and Hitch were still there and painful!

I went in and Patrick suggested that I stop my workouts for a few weeks and let his Symmetry process start working. Not wanting to really stop my progress for my race training, I was very skeptical, but I decided to "Get Better" and to listen to my body yelling at me so I stopped my workouts for a couple of weeks.

About 1 ½ months into faithfully doing the individualized routines that Patrick set up for me, I had my Spartan Sprint Race. During the race, I was completing an obstacle that normally had my hip in an upset. I was feeling like something was missing and realized it was the intense pain! The pain level was greatly diminished.

Fast forward 4 months and 5 races later, my hip has no pain. My running time actually went down since my legs and hips can move the proper way, with no "hitch" in my step. And another added bonus, my pinky and index fingers no longer fall asleep. In the past I went to my doctor and they wanted to do surgery to help with the fingers falling asleep and tingling I was experiencing. After going through Symmetry, I am happy to say I haven't had any sleeping fingers or tingling.

Walking into Symmetry is always a wonderful experience for me. I love all the staff and they have all been extremely helpful. I highly suggest that you see them and see how they can help you!"

Crystal

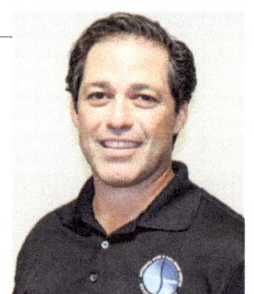

"My name is Andrew Bloch. Amongst other things, I am a Physical Therapist as well as a licensed Acupuncturist. I met Patrick 3 years ago at a symposium in San Diego. I remember distinctly walking by his booth and seeing his system of corrective exercises up on his 44" flat screen. I gravitated immediately to Patrick's product because I just listened to a conference on qualitative postural analysis which left me wanting something different to help me identify potential postural dysfunction. As Patrick began to explain to me how he had created an entire patented system of corrective exercises through measuring posture and creating a quantifiable report to not only explain his treatment protocols, but verify and validate them from session to session, I was very impressed. This type of advanced technology is sorely missing in the Physical Technology world. Four months later my business partner, Dr. Brian Paris, and I flew Patrick out to take our clinic through his certification program.

For four years now, we have utilized the AlignSmart™ system in our office. Not only does it validate our evaluations for insurance, but more importantly validates the treatments I use for my patients. Using Reflexive Pattern Technology™, a system that I created for immediate pain relief, I then have an incredible postural measurement report each session along with the corrective exercise portion of the AlignSmart system, which allows the added benefit of my treatments to hold for a much longer period of time. Also, the emphasis is now transferred to my patients to become proactive in their own treatment by knowing exactly what to do on their own in between their visits with me!

As a healthcare practitioner, both traditional and non-traditional, it is imperative that practitioner's move from qualitative to quantitative data and then use this data to allow a client to be involved in the process of getting well. Symmetry's AlignSmart™ technology is the wave of the future, so catch it now and don't be left behind."

Andrew Bloch, MSPT, L.Ac.,
President - Advanced Spine & Wellness Center
Creator of Reflexive Pattern Technology™

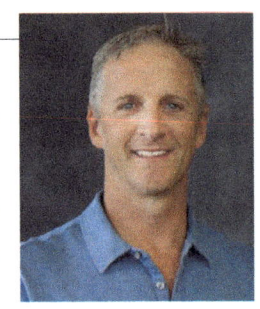

"In over 27 years as a Chiropractic wellness provider I have been exposed to many different forms of spinal exercise and gimmicks relative to spinal recovery and rehabilitation. Some of those methods are useful and effective, and I routinely use elements of these approaches as an aspect of our spinal corrective protocols. In 2014 I was exposed to a new systematic approach to postural correction called "Symmetry for Health". I was intrigued as one of my stubborn, chronic pain clients had recently received great results from this approach. As is customary for me I decided to check it out for myself from a patient's perspective. As a new client, I was very impressed by the technology behind their assessment and was even more impressed by the results I achieved with the unique, specific rehab protocols they suggested for me. I love that it is mostly self-guided and feel their web based platform is revolutionary for the rehab and postural correction industry.

I routinely refer my clients to "Symmetry for Health" as a way to effectively balance and strengthen their body so ultimately, they hold the corrective adjustments we perform on them. If you are not holding your adjustments and are looking for an approach that is corrective and effective, you must check out "Symmetry for Health"."

Dr. Ron Simms, D.C., CEO of Back to Health Chiropractic

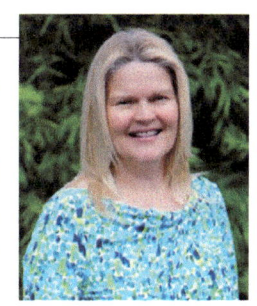

"I've known Patrick for over 15 years when a colleague recommended I see him for back pain. My surgeon friend had a slipped disc that was referred for surgery. After participating in Symmetry not only was my friend back in the OR but he was skiing within 6 months! Although my back pain was not as bad, I had pain with every day activities like driving, bending over to examine patients and sitting at my computer. After 3 sessions with Patrick my pain was gone and I was able to participate in my first sprint triathlon within 4 months - pain free! His postural alignment theories, assessments and exercise program make sense and work well. I've trusted Symmetry to help many family, friends and colleagues that I have referred over the years."

Linda Smith, M.D., FAAP

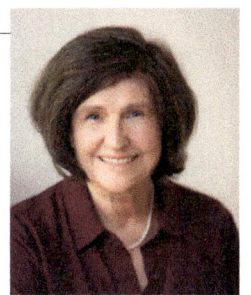

"Patrick mummy relieved my pain when I first came to him. In addition, I also saw a huge increase in my strength, so I could tolerate the exercises I wanted in my life, such as walks and ballroom dancing. Out of my holistic medical practice, I refer a lot of patients for Symmetry work who have had VERY quick relief of their pain. I think the work that Patrick Mummy does has accurate bio mechanics and physics as its basis, and out of that can really give people an individualized program that supports their strengthening over time. It also is extremely complementary to any individual body work they might have like chiropractic, massage or cranial sacral which can be temporary, momentary treatments. The person has control of **his/her** own improvements daily to correct their structure, maintain strength and achieve their personal physical goals! I would not hesitate to recommend this program."

Kelly Sutton, MD, Raphael Medicine + Therapies, PC

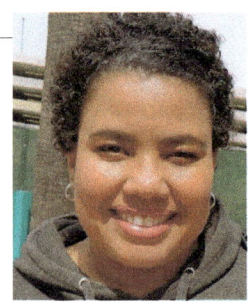

"I found Symmetry when I was at an all-time low. We were a year into the Great Recession and my back went out. This would be manageable except that doing massages and running my small three-room massage clinic now looked like an impossibility.

Somehow, amid my tears, fears and anger, my dear friend Angie managed to calm me down. She put me on the floor and took me through two Symmetry™ exercises that immediately took my back pain away.

I was stunned.

That night I kept looking for and expecting the pain to return… but it just didn't. I knew I had to know more about Symmetry™ so I looked online and began a journey that night that I'll be forever thankful I started.

Once I looked deeper, I decided I needed to schedule an appointment with Patrick to go through the full Symmetry™ experience. I'll never forget him laughing at my pain and telling me he didn't care – and he was right! I'd been trained for my entire career to "chase the pain" but never to get to the root of it and correct the cause.

The AlignSmart™ system does this and so much more. I have

never found a more complete system of health care than what Patrick has created. Not only did I receive compassionate and educated care, I learned how to take care of my own body in a totally new and empowering way.

Symmetry has taught me that I don't need to suffer. That growing older doesn't mean accepting aches and pains as a way of life. It's taught me that I can literally control how I feel on any given day. For this and more, I am eternally grateful.

Once I stopped being a Symmetry patient, I knew I needed to become a practitioner.

Over the course of my five-year journey to becoming a Certified Level 3 practitioner, I've personally witnessed amazing transformations in people that have literally changed their lives - from massage therapists finally having that 'Aha' moment to Physical Therapists and Acupuncturists getting excited again about caring for their patients. Seeing their renewed joy at being able to actually provide health care again only fueled my passion for this work.

As a practitioner, I've seen people break down in tears in front of me from sheer relief. Ten years of pain vanishing in a few minutes is truly the norm with this work.

Patrick's generous and loving nature is infused in this work- his demeanor cannot be separated from the work he does. I believe that this is what takes Symmetry above simply being another health care modality to being a complete health care system.

In my mind, I can give no higher recommendation than that. Do this and you'll experience love. Love for your body, love for the work and love for sharing it with others. Being able to help the people we love is a universal desire at the root of our nature. With Symmetry, you'll be able to do that and more."

Angel Martinez, CMT, SPP

Symmetry prevented me from getting back surgery - 18 years ago!

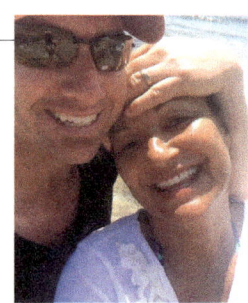

"In 2000 a friend of mine convinced me to go see someone by the name of Patrick who owned a business called "Symmetry." My friend was very uncomfortable with my impending surgery - especially knowing there was a better answer for me. Well, since I figured I had nothing to lose I thought I would give Symmetry a try.

It took me almost two hours to go through the initial routine as I was in excruciating pain. I had also been on pain management medication for about a year. The thing that struck me about Patrick's approach was that it all made sense and no one had ever mentioned the connection between my posture or lack of good posture and the constant pain I had been having. Not to mention Patrick's gentle yet firm manner.

Imagine my surprise when later that evening I was crouching on the floor playing with my two cats. It was then that I suddenly realized that I was no longer in pain - no pain - no discomfort - completely able to move for the first time in several years! I had thought that my life was never going to be the same. That I was never going to be able to surf or swim or run around with my children. This program was so effective that within two short weeks I began to believe that I was going to have a full and active life once again - that it really was possible and that I was actually living that possibility. I cancelled the surgery and have NEVER looked back. It's been 18 years.

It was so effective that Executives at my company, peoplefirst.com noticed right away that something was different. They had bought me a sciatic desk chair at a cost of $2000 to help relieve my pain. Dave, the COO had chronic knee problems for years - it worked for him, then he introduced Symmetry to his wife, it worked for her, then he spoke with Gary the CEO and decided to offer it to all of the employees in the company. That's how effective Symmetry was and is for everyone.

I have now been doing Patrick's Symmetry routines for the last 18 years. It has been such an effective and successful program for me that I finally decided to marry him - at least that way I could get the technology for free! In all seriousness - try this program. Try this program if you've ever been told that surgery is the only option, or that there just isn't any help for you. Try this program if you want to be a faster more effective athlete. Try this program if you just want to grow older more gracefully. Just give it a chance - I'm living, active proof that it works!

Tricia Mummy, wife.